To Live Without Pain

The Way to Reduce, Prevent and Suppress
Back & Spinal Pain

Author:
Dr. Ronen Welgrin, D.C.

The Best Methods
for Natural Self-Healing
and to Improve Well-being

This is certainly a must-read book for anyone
who wants to enjoy a life free from back pain

Dr. Ronen Welgrin

To Live Without Pain

Images: Gonen Shemer
Cover and book design: Studio Lev Ari
Translation: Tip Top Translations

To Live Without Pain

The Way to Prevent, Reduce and Suppress
Back & Spinal Pain

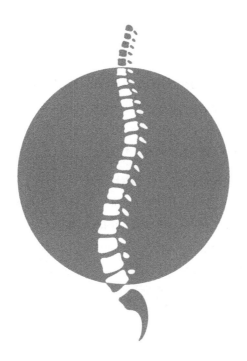

The reference in masculine text as written in the book is for
convenience purposes only.
The book addresses both genders.

Table of Contents

Thanks 9

Clarification. 10

About the Author 12

Introduction 14

How to Maximize Your Benefit From This Book? 18

Why Did I Write This Book?. 20

Chapter One: Life Without Pain 23

"First and Foremost ....Health"! 25
- Health, Luck or Money - What is More Important? 25
- Have You Heard of Spinal Transplants? 28
- Does a Lack of Back Pain Necessarily Mean
  That You Are Healthy? 30

Chapter Two: The Spine - Basic Concepts 33
- Structure of the Spine 35
- Curves are Not Always a Negative Thing About Spinal Curves 40
- The Functions of the Spine 43
- The Importance of the Pelvis 44

**Chapter Three: The Importance
of the Nervous System** 47
Nerves - The Most Important Wiring System You Will Ever Know! 49

Chapter Four: Should Problems Start, Consult your Physician 53

- Getting to the Root of the Problem: Reasons and Problems that Cause Neck, Back and Spinal Pain 55
- What is My Spine Trying to Tell Me? Symptoms that May Occur Due to Spinal Problems 60
- Doctor, Do I Have a Back Problem? 68
- I Have a Back Problem, What Should I Do? 69
- When to Seek Urgent Medical Help? 71

Chapter Five: Solutions Revealed 73

Correct Posture 75

- The Importance of Learning Correct Posture to Prevent Spinal Impairments 75
- Six Ways to Detect Spinal Impairments with a Posture Test . . 78
- Potential Damage Due to the Incorrect Position of the Head and Neck. 83
- Possible Damages Caused by Prolonged Bending of the Middle Back 86
- My Grandfather's Posture at the Age of 100! 89
- The Natural Curves of My Spine are Almost Unnoticeable. Is that Good? 92
- Learn How to Overcome an Exaggerated Lumbar Curve 95

Standing 99

- Learn How to Reduce and Even Prevent Back Pain While Standing. 99
- Learn to Work with your Body Close to Objects. 103
- Introducing – The 'Sumo Stance'. 105
- Learn to Work with Your Body Facing Objects 107
- Push or Pull – Which is Best? 109
- Knee Bending as a Method to Prevent and Reduce the Risk of Back Pain 112

- Learn to Minimize Forward Inclination of the Torso
  or Bending Your Torso While Standing 114
- Learn How to Prevent or Reduce Back Pain in the Gym. . . . 116

Lifting and Putting Down Objects. 118
- The Correct Order of Movement to Prevent Back Damage . 118
- My Grandparents' Pulley 122
- Which Object Should be Picked Up First? 123
- How to Reduce or Prevent Back Pain While Placing
  Your Infant in a Car? 125

Symmetry: Use Both Sides of the Body 127
- Preventing Back Problems with Symmetrical Effort 127
- Recommended Places to Sit
  in a Banquet Hall 130
- The Common Mistake of Amateur Swimmers,
  Swimming the Front Crawl Stroke 132

Sitting 134
- The Negative Effects Prolonged Sitting Has on the Body . . . 134
- The Negative Effects Prolonged Sitting has on the Back . . . 136
- Learn to Reduce Your Sitting Time 138
- Try to Sit Straight and Not Slouch 140
- The Effect Electric Bicycles have on Backs 142
- Use Lower Back Support to Reduce and Prevent Pain 143
- Learn to Use Your Hands While Sitting to Avoid Back Pain. . 144
- Learn How to Reduce Back Pain While Sitting on a Sofa . . . 146
- In Which Pocket Should you Keep your Wallet? 150
- Learn to Minimize Lifting Objects While Sitting 151
- How to Get Up from a Chair Without Damaging your Back?. 153
- Correct Bathroom Posture is Important 157

How to Behave with a Disc Problem? 159
- Learn About One of the Main Reasons
  of Various Disc Problems 159

- How to Put Shoes on and Tie Laces, Even When Suffering from a Protruding or Herniated Disc?. 164
- Recommended Seats During a Flight for Those Suffering from a Protruding or Herniated Disc 167
- How to Get Into Bed Without Pain? 169
- Traction or Compression? Methods for Treating Problematic Discs 171

Lying Down 172
- How to Reduce and Prevent Back Pain While Lying Down? . 172
- Secrets from the Bedroom. 176

The Effect of Obesity on Back Pain 178

The Effect Coughing or Sneezing Has on Pain Levels . . . 180

Sporting Activities 182
- How to Maintain Strong Back Vertebrae? 182
- Optimal Spinal Motion Range 185
- Learn the Importance of Abdominal Muscles 188
- Know How to Strengthen Your Back Muscles 193
- Learn How to Strengthen Your Leg Muscles to Avoid Back Pain 197

Epilogue 198

Please Note!

The material contained in this book is based on the best medical knowledge available today. However, this book is not intended as a substitute for medical advice or medical treatment, and its purpose is to provide the reader with general knowledge only. The reader should consult his / her physician on a regular basis in all matters related to his / her health, including any significant change in his / her health. Do not use the different treatment methods and tips written in this book without medical advice. The author is not responsible for any damage that may be caused by the use of the information contained in this book, and rejects any claim in advance.

Thanks

I would like to thank my father, Michael Welgrin, who helped me realize many dreams throughout my life and who supported me without limits.

To my dear wife Ilana, for her infinite love, support and giving.

To my dear children Yuval, Inbar and Harel - I love you all.

To my family, my acquaintances, and all my patients who inspired my writing and who offered their good advice.

Clarification

This book was written to help you learn and understand **how to prevent, reduce** and even **suppress back pain**. After more than twenty years of helping thousands of people, both in my clinic and by giving lectures to the general public, offering valuable information on the subject, I understood that there are different ways and actions that, if implemented, are able to prevent back pain. Actions that significantly relieve pain, and of course, prevent the recurrence of problems to those who previously had suffered with this condition.

For years, I have consistently practiced these exercises to prevent my own spinal damage. The actions and exercises described in the book allow me to enjoy a life free from back pain and to become a role model for thousands of people interested in living a life without back pain. The spinal condition and quality of life of many children, adults, and senior citizens who have acted on my guidance and advice has significantly improved.

This book does not deal with taking forms of medication, injections or undergoing surgery, but rather, actions that benefit the body and behavior patterns. If you carry out these actions, they can help you maintain a healthy back, save you from pain and thus improve your quality of your life.

No one can guarantee an immediate improvement in your condition or your pain level. Sometimes there is irreversible damage caused to the back and spine that cannot be solved, and sometimes there are complex, chronic problems that persist for many years and whose treatment is not successful. However, your strict adherence to proper body posture and movement on a **daily basis** and performing the exercises described in this book, **regularly and over time**, can improve your condition, even if there is irreversible damage or you suffer from chronic problems.

I highly recommend consulting with a medical professional regarding your general health condition, and your back and spine in particular.

I hope that this book will help you prevent back problems, reduce and even eliminate pain that already exists, to improve your quality of life.

I would like to take this opportunity to thank you for purchasing this book. I would be happy to hear your feedback, comments, remarks and observations. If you believe that this book may help other people, I would appreciate it if you would recommend this book to them.

About the Author

Dr. Ronen Welgrin is a well-known chiropractor[1] and lecturer in the field of posture, spine, neck, and back health. During his lectures, he provides **valuable knowledge** that helps the audience prevent, reduce, and even significantly improve existing neck, back and spinal problems or those that may be caused in the future. He also explains how to prevent and minimize **other body problems that are often caused** due to spinal problems and can result in headaches, pain, numbness, and 'shooting pains' in hands and feet.

Dr. Welgrin successfully graduated as a Chiropractor in 1997 from the prestigious Logan College in St. Louis, Missouri, USA.

He is an active member of the Israel Chiropractic Association and holds the necessary permits to work in his field on behalf of the Israeli Ministry of Health.

Additionally, he participates in Israel's professional courses and seminars, has over 20 years' experience in a wide range of spine, back and neck problems and has run a private clinic in Israel for many years.

---

1 Chiropractic is a medical health profession that focuses on diagnosing, treating and preventing neurological, musculoskeletal, and skeletal disorders, and the effects of these deficiencies on general health. Chiropractic refers to the spine as a significant factor that affects human health. Those practicing chiropractic implement many treatment methods, used worldwide to assist in a wide range of neck, joint and limb problems, back pain, headaches and more.

Dr. Welgrin helps thousands of people with spinal, back and neck problems. He provides professional services to large entities, such as leading insurance companies and the Ministry of Defense, through which he has treated disabled veterans of the Israel Defense Forces and the Ministry of Rehabilitation, for many years.

In 2004, he was chosen as an outstanding employee at Clalit Health Services Complementary Medicine clinic, where he has been involved with since 1998.

Dr. Welgrin is also a graduate of the Wingate Institute where, in 1992, he completed his studies in physical education for schools. In the course of his studies, he specialized in **promoting** good **posture** and **preventative exercise**, identifying posture impairments in children such as scoliosis, kyphosis (humpback), and hyperlordosis (increased lumbar curvature) alongside additional conditions, and methods of treating these impairments.

Dr. Welgrin is a sports enthusiast who regularly engages in physical activity. He is a certified gym instructor and lifeguard. He is married to Ilana, and together they raise their three children, Yuval, Inbar and Harel.

Dr. Welgrin aims to spread his knowledge, making it accessible to as many people as possible, in order to improve their health.

Those interested in lectures or personal counseling in his fields of expertise are welcome to contact him via email: ronenwelgrin@gmail.com or call his cellular phone +972-54-4626196.

Introduction

"Ronen, come and help me!" were the words my mother cried out from her bedroom, where she had been taking a nap. It happened one day back in 1976, and I was a nine-year-old boy in the middle of doing my homework.

I ran to her room. Her call was urgent, and I could tell by her tone of voice that she needed immediate help. When I got to her room, I saw her struggling to get up from her bed, while complaining that her back hurt.

I tried to help her to the best of my ability but she was in so much pain, there was nothing I could do. After several attempts, my mother managed to sit on the bed. Her complaints about lower back pain continued for a long time after, but the doctors found no effective remedy or treatment to help her. My parents continued to consult with other doctors. My mother was prescribed even stronger painkillers but sadly, her condition did not improve. The pain was continuous, and later the doctors decided to put her in a plaster cast, with the thought that perhaps, by immobilizing her back, her pain would ease.

My mother's condition was deteriorating.

I remember a picture of my mother lying in the hospital in her plaster cast, helping me prepare for an exam that I was supposed to have in the next few days. She wrote questions on a piece of paper; her handwriting was shaky and although her health continued to deteriorate, she struggled to help me as much as she could.

My mother passed away from cancer on November 2, 1977 at the age of 34. The picture of her lying in that hospital bed with her plaster cast will be engraved in my memory forever.

That was my first acquaintance with back pain.

My father later told me that during our period of mourning, I used to tell the people who came to console us that, "When I grow up, I will help people be healthier." I have been trying to fulfill these words for many years, both in my clinic and in lectures to different audiences, to provide knowledge and share the expertise I have gained from many years of study. So far, I have had the privilege of helping literally thousands of people with my recommendations and advice, and I hope that this book can help you, relieve your pain, prevent new problems and pave the way for a happy and healthy life.

After my mother passed away, my childhood was uneventful. Upon completing my national service, my great love for physical activity led to a four-year course in physical education at the Wingate Institute in Israel.

This was my first in-depth study of the human body and the functioning of its different systems. I specialized in **promoting good** posture and **preventative exercise**, and my studies provided me with deep insights in spine, neck and back issues.

This knowledge enabled me to treat children in schools with various posture impairments such as scoliosis, kyphosis, hyperlordosis, and other problems. I did this through physical activity such as exercises to strengthen and stretch certain muscles, posture exercises, etc.

This basic and necessary knowledge enabled me to provide advice to people about back health and how to improve their well-being. The subject of physical health continued to interest and fascinate me. I felt that I had to increase my depth of knowledge in order to provide a better medical response to people. I decided to continue my studies and went on to study Chiropractic at St. Louis, Missouri, United States.

The many medical subjects I have studied over the years such as anatomy, dissection, x-ray, pathology, orthopedics, neurology, kinesiology, and many other subjects, have all greatly contributed in enriching my knowledge of health and enabled me to treat, direct and guide people towards improving their health, well-being and to enjoy a better quality of life.

The knowledge and experiences I have acquired have also helped me save lives. I saved my nephew from choking on a foreign body and losing consciousness when he was just four years old! I have also helped many others with neck, back, muscle and skeletal problems such as disc herniation, joint degeneration, shoulder and knee problems, chronic and acute pain, mobility issues, etc.

The way you treat your back and maintain your spine in optimum condition, alongside maintaining your overall health, can help you enjoy a better quality of life and live with less pain.

Dear Reader, I hope that you live to a good old age with good health, which will allow you to travel, visit and explore new places under your own steam and free of back pain!

After many years of accumulating theoretical and practical knowledge, I have written this book with much excitement and enthusiasm, and I truly hope that you will benefit from reading its contents.

Recently, I had the opportunity to successfully treat someone who knew my family and my mother, and he confirmed that he had indeed heard my childhood vision to help people, following my mother's death, more than forty years ago.

I wish you good health,
Dr. Ronen Welgrin
Chiropractor

How to Maximize Your Benefit From This Book?

This book contains various patterns of action and behavior that I have personally been using for years to successfully maintain the health of my back. Since the health of your spine, back and neck depends on a **sequence of correct actions, they should be carried out as frequently and as long as possible, on a daily basis**. I recommend that you read the book from beginning to end, without skipping pages, to ensure you will not miss out any important tips that can help you.

Suppose, for example, that you experience pain while sitting due to a disc problem. You will probably want to refer to and read the section on how to reduce pain while sitting. However, if you do not know how to correct your posture while standing up, washing your face in the morning, lifting a bag off the floor and getting into your car correctly, then it will be more difficult to reduce the pain you experience while sitting.

Your main goal should be to **accomplish as many correct actions as possible on a daily basis** in order to maximize your chances of improving the health of your back and spine. Therefore, I strongly recommend that you do not skip pages, and as soon as you notice important sentences, mark them with a pencil at the side of the page so that you can quickly return to them for future reference.

Additionally, since this book contains a lot of information on the subject, it is likely that you will not remember the various insights listed in it. Re-reading the book may help you to remember the different courses of action recommended, thus increasing your chances of actually implementing the exercises later on.

I am delighted that you have taken this book into your hands and are reading these lines, and I greatly appreciate your desire to learn about and improve the health of your spine and back.

Why Did I Write This Book?

During my many years of work, I have noticed how children, youth, adults, and the elderly put their back and spinal health at risk. Their posture, the way they incorrectly sit, walk, lie down and perform simple daily tasks such as washing their face in the morning, lifting a bag, sitting at a table and even getting into the car, can cause damage to their spine. I found myself constantly guiding, correcting and teaching my patients, my family, my acquaintances, and my friends, the way to keep a healthy back. Although some of them had no pain at all, I recognized significant mistakes in how they functioned with their spine and I knew they were unaware that they were doing harm to themselves. Most of them had chronic back and spine problems, which were accompanied by functional problems and a real impairment in their quality of life.

I considered how much pain and suffering they could spare themselves if they would function correctly with their spine. Obviously, I tried to help them as best I could, and yet I realized that this contribution was only beneficial to the people with whom I was in direct contact. I tried to think of a way I could help many people around the world improve their quality of life and live their lives free of back pain. I noticed that many back problems began at an early age, and if I did not teach adults how to function correctly, how would they ever have the skills to teach their children, and even take care of their own health?

Many people experience back and neck problems; they do not know how incorrect posture affects their bodies. Sometimes it is due to lack of knowledge on the subject, sometimes due to laziness, sometimes due to incorrect guidance, and sometimes due to body problems and pains. These reasons cause them to repeatedly make the same mistakes. Therefore, is it any wonder that their situation does not improve?

This book was written with the intention of providing as many people as possible, no matter their age, with tools to help them improve their quality of life. Over the years, I have repeatedly heard the disappointment and frustration of many people who suffer from back problems. Some find it difficult to sit at work or even at home, some are afraid to travel because of the pain they experience, some suffer pain when lifting small children, and many others experience hours of pain on a daily basis, which makes their daily routine or living in general an unpleasant experience.

Many people who have heard my lectures, along with many of my patients, have asked me for written information about the various exercises and methods I use which allow me to personally enjoy a life free of back pain.

I am very happy that I have succeeded in writing this book for you and hope that your perseverance and practice will lead you to enjoy a better quality of life and optimal functioning, pain free!

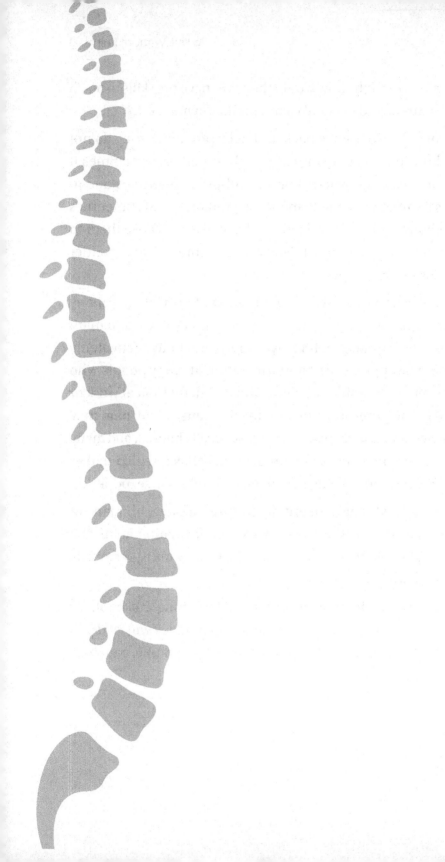

Chapter One

Life Without Pain

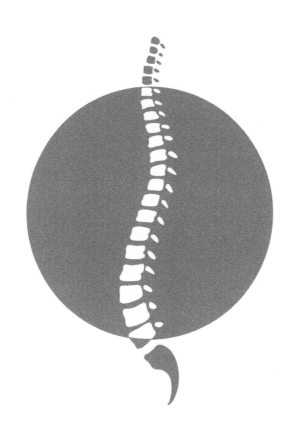

"First and Foremost ....Health"!

Health, Luck or Money - What is More Important?

I would like to ask you a question. What is important to you in life? A relationship? Livelihood? Money? Love? Family? Maybe additional values or a combination of some of those mentioned. What do you think is the order of priorities for most people?

My father, a man with a great deal of life experience, became a widower at a very young age. As I have already told you, my mother died at the age of just thirty-four after suffering from a serious illness. My father was forced to cope with the raising of his three small children and to take care of all their needs. Although he got help from our immediate family, and even from a nanny, the responsibility that lay on his shoulders was still immense. Despite all this, my father tried to support, guide and direct us, so that we would not feel any different from other children. I remember my father working days and nights just to support us, and his determination to succeed and raise a wonderful family was admirable.

My father had to start his life anew in his thirties, and his outlook of life changed. When I asked him, "Dad, what is the most important thing in life?" he would reply, "First of all, health." When I asked him what else was important in life, he would reply, "Luck and money."

Today, after many years of helping patients in my clinic, my father's insights are even clearer to me. Sometimes people come to the clinic and say, "Tell me how much money the treatments are going to cost me to make me well" Unfortunately, in medicine, in my field of work which deals with spinal health, money is not always the solution. I often encounter cases of irreversible damage due to patients' lack of implementing therapeutic recommendations they have received. Therefore, we must constantly act to maintain our health, and not to neglect it. Health is first and foremost!

The term 'luck' is not as specific as health and money and may actually be expressed in every aspect of our lives. It is difficult to define, but I would say, in my experience, that it is the talent to seize a good opportunity at the right time or be in the right place at the right time. For example, a lucky patient is one who comes to me for to a series of treatments based on a friend's recommendation, literally just before surgery, and by doing so avoids the surgery completely.

I totally agree with my father who chose health first, followed by luck and money. This is exactly the right order. Firstly, be healthy and look after your health. Then you should try to be lucky, being aware of opportunities that occur such as being in the right place at the right time (it depends a bit on you and a little on fate), and finally, money also never hurts.

This book deals with the spine and back, as stated. As I will explain below, I believe that keeping the spine functioning and maintaining your spine on a daily basis will allow you to be healthier and enjoy a better quality of life. As for luck and money? I will leave that to you.

Have You Heard of Spinal Transplants?

The human body is one of the most complex machines known to man.

It consists of various systems that affect our body 24 hours a day, such as the respiratory, digestive and nervous systems. Proper functioning of the various organs of the body is vitally important for optimal health. There are situations in which, due to trauma such as a car accident, an injury, a fall or even an illness, the damaged organ needs to be replaced by a new organ.

Organ transplants began in the 1950s and 1960s. For the first time, a heart, kidney, lung and liver were transplanted. Today these organ transplants are performed successfully in many countries around the world. However, in those days, spinal transplants were not performed. There was considerable difficulty in how to deal with the spinal cord and the nerves that emerge from it. Medical science continued to progress, and in the early 2000s, facial transplants, limb transplants, uterine transplants and many others were successfully performed.

The spine is one of the biggest challenges in transplants.

In 2014, a team of surgeons in Beijing, China, under the direction of Dr. Liu Zhongjun, the head of the hospital's orthopedic department, succeeded in transplanting a printed three-dimensional vertebra in the neck of a 12-year-old boy. This is probably the first use of a printed vertebrae implant, in spinal surgery.

In October 2014, a Bulgarian man was reported to have started walking after being paralyzed from the waist down. Doctors from the University College of London, directed by Professor Geoffrey Riesman, took nerve cells from the patient's nose. After being grown in the laboratory, the cells were implanted by Polish surgeons, headed by Dr. Pavel Tabakov, in the patient's spinal cord. The damaged nerve ends from the damaged tissues in the patient's back began to grow, and after two years of exercises and training, the man began to slowly walk.

Hopefully, this groundbreaking study will help those suffering spinal cord injuries and pave the way for their full rehabilitation. Many people fail to maintain the health of their back. Most people are not aware of proper posture, and their knowledge in maintaining a healthy back is minimal. Therefore, it is no wonder that many people suffer, and some even need surgery.

A supreme effort in public education must be made regarding maintaining a healthy back and maintaining proper posture from an early age, in order to prevent future back problems for people as they grow older.

I hope that the information in this book will help you maintain the health of your back and enjoy a happy and healthy life.

Remember! Most organs in the human body can be replaced, except for the spine and nerves that pass through and emerge from it. Therefore, look after your spine, because it has no substitute!

Does a Lack of Back Pain Necessarily Mean That You Are Healthy?

Some people think that the appearance or non-appearance of pain is the only measure to determine a person's health. Are they right? Is the assumption 'Nothing hurts me, so I am healthy' correct? Does lack of back pain definitively mean that the spine is in normal condition? To answer these questions, I will use a few examples.

The first example, hypertension, is known as the 'silent killer'. Many people walk around with no complaint or pain. They feel healthy and think they are in good condition, cardiac-wise. However, it is a fact that some of those with prolonged, undiagnosed, and untreated hypertension have an increased chance of having a heart attack or stroke, even though they feel fine, without any complaints. Even if a person feels in good health and has no pain, he should regularly monitor his blood pressure. By doing so and taking medication if necessary, one can reduce mortality rates.

Another example is high blood glucose levels that are present in diabetes. We know that various organs, such as the eyes and kidneys, can be damaged as a result of diabetes that has been undiagnosed or is not controlled optimally even when no pain is felt. Here too, early diagnosis of the disease through a simple blood test can save a lot of future suffering.

The latest example is from dentistry. Brushing, flossing, and periodic tartar removal are some of the recommended actions to prevent future pain and oral problems.

I guess you have gotten the message. Examination of your spine and back by a chiropractor or any other professional is essential to prevent future irreversible damage to your body. Periodic examination by a chiropractor, which may be accompanied by an X-ray if necessary, may detect spinal abnormalities such as scoliosis, kyphosis (humpback), vertebral misalignment, disc problems, nerve compression, etc.

The absence of back pain or lack of complaint of any back problems does not necessarily indicate a good state of health.

This book contains many tips on how to prevent, reduce and even eliminate back pain. Even if you do not feel any pain, it is recommended that you read the book, acquire the proper knowledge and apply it in practice to prevent pain and problems in the future.

In conclusion, do not wait for pain to get your back checked! Pain appears after the damage has already been done! Get your spine checked as soon as possible - and from time to time - to prevent and spare yourself future problems.

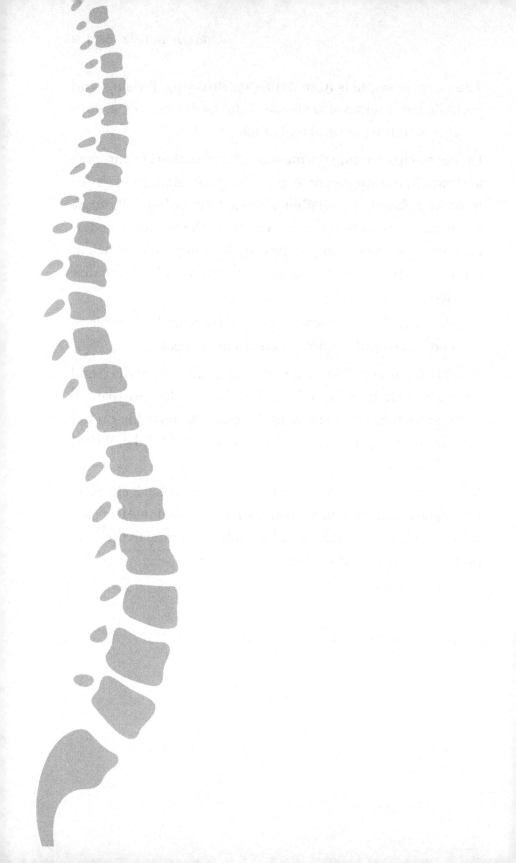

Chapter Two

The Spine -
Basic Concepts

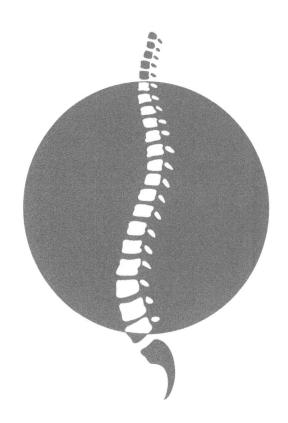

Structure of the Spine

The spine consists of 32-34 vertebrae and starts from the base of the skull in the occipital bone, forming a bilateral joint with the first cervical vertebra, and descends down to the tailbone (coccyx). See Figure 1 below.

The spine can be divided into several sections, from the top down:

- The cervical section consists of 7 vertebrae.

- The thoracic section (chest) consists of 12 vertebrae.

- The lumbar section consists of 5 vertebrae.

- The sacrum consists of 5 vertebrae that have fused.

- The coccyx or the 'tailbone' consists of 3 to 5 vertebrae that have fused.

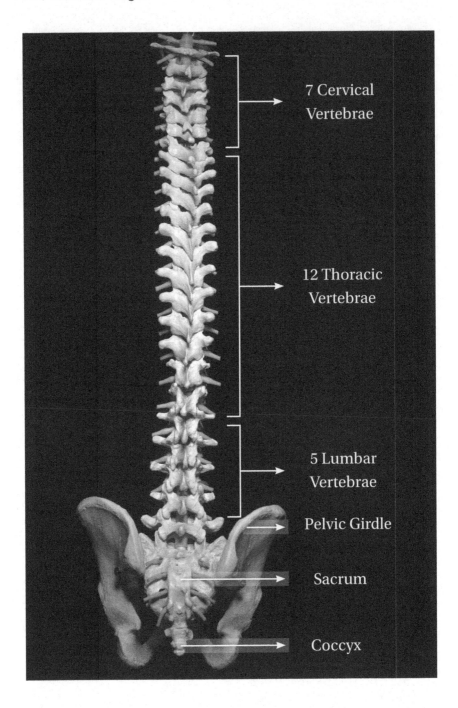

Figure 1: A Plastic Model of the Spinal Column - Rear View

From the second cervical vertebra downwards, between each two vertebrae, there is a **disc** or cartilage serves as a shock absorber. If the disc or cartilage is in proper condition, it prevents the contact and compression of two adjacent vertebrae. See Figure 2 below. The cervical, thoracic, and lumbar vertebrae, except for the first two vertebrae in the neck, are quite similar in terms of the parts that form each vertebra. It is also possible to see similarity in the shape of these vertebrae.

In general, the front part of the vertebra which faces towards the abdomen, is called the **vertebral body**. The vertebral body is bigger as it reaches the lower back in order to be able to carry the increased weight of the body. Behind the vertebral body is the vertebral canal which is enclosed by the back of the vertebra in the form of an arched structure called the **vertebral arch** or the **neural arch.** Within this cavity is the spinal cord. When the vertebrae are placed on top of each other, they form a long channel through which the spinal cord passes, called the spinal canal. A side view between any two adjacent vertebrae, will show you a kind of oval-shaped cavity. The spinal nerve passes through this cavity behind the bodies of those vertebrae. **This space is called the Foraminal Canal or the intervertebral foramen.**

Bony processes extend from the vertebral arch in different directions, which form points of connection to the muscles and tendons. **Two upper joint surfaces and two lower joint surfaces** also extend from the vertebral arch, which enable movement and articulation of the vertebrae.

The cervical vertebrae have a unique characteristic in the appearance of a small circular cavity within their transverse process, through which the artery of the vertebrae goes up to the head and is responsible for some of the blood supply to the brain. The thoracic vertebrae create joints to connect with the ribs, thus enabling breathing. The lumbar vertebrae are larger than the cervical and thoracic vertebrae, allowing them to carry body weight. Beneath the lumbar vertebrae is a fused bone, the sacrum, which is similar in shape to a triangle and forms the upper back wall of the pelvic cavity. This bone consists of the fusion of five bones and has openings through which nerves emerge. The sacrum creates joints with the last lumbar vertebrae above, with the pelvic bones on either side and with the coccyx below. The coccyx is the lowest part of the spine.

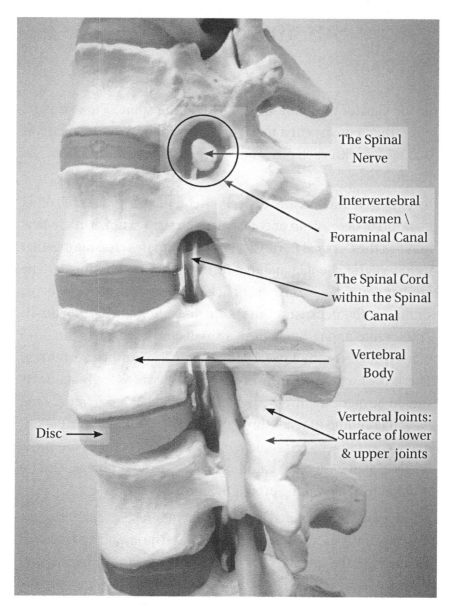

The Spinal Nerve

Intervertebral Foramen \ Foraminal Canal

The Spinal Cord within the Spinal Canal

Vertebral Body

Vertebral Joints: Surface of lower & upper joints

Disc

Figure 2: A side view of a plastic model demonstrating several lumbar vertebrae

Curves are Not Always a Negative Thing About Spinal Curves

A side view of the spine will show that the spine is not straight, but rather, consists of a number of inward and outward curves that merge with each other and form an S-shaped structure. See Figure 3 below.

In normal conditions, the cervical vertebrae lay on top of each other in a kind of depression or concaved arch shape known in medical terms as **the Cervical Lordosis.** The dorsal spine vertebrae together form a slightly bent shape that forms the **Dorsal Kyphosis.** The lumbar vertebrae in the lower back form a concaved arch shape, similar to the neck vertebrae, known as the **Lumbar Lordosis.** The sacrum and tailbone form a small convex shape in the form of a **kyphosis in the lowest area below the lumbar vertebrae.** This is the **normal position** of the spinal curves, and **great efforts** should be made to prevent their enlargement or reduction in size. As you continue to read through the book, you will learn about many cases in which a change in the natural curves of the spine is associated with back pain problems. These problems can be avoided by maintaining proper posture.

Spinal curves are affected by several factors such as genetics, age, poor posture, various diseases and injuries. The inward and outward directions of the spinal curves, allow the spine to absorb loads and shocks that are applied to it more effectively, thereby minimizing the chance of back and neck problems. Activities such as running, jumping and walking with a backpack, create mechanical loads on the vertebrae. If the spine was straight, it would be more susceptible to damage from these normal activities.

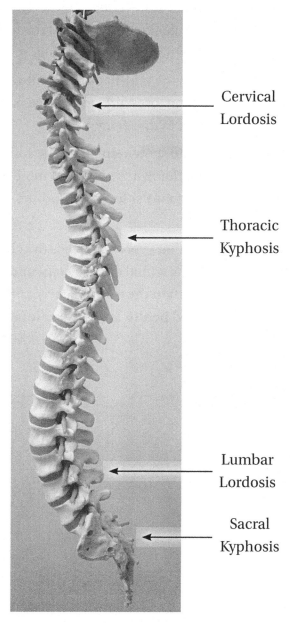

Cervical
Lordosis

Thoracic
Kyphosis

Lumbar
Lordosis

Sacral
Kyphosis

Figure 3: A plastic model of the spine – side view

Decreasing spinal curves cause movement limitation and increase pressure on the back, neck and pelvis. This leads to phenomena such as pain, degenerative changes and dysfunction in various daily activities, which affect well-being.

Increasing spinal curves in the mid-back and lumbar areas, for example, can cause back pain, pressure on internal organs, and later on, abnormal function of these organs.

A rear view of the spine should show a straight spine and deviation of the vertebrae from their natural place, in one or more segments, expressed by their rotation and sideward bending, known as scoliosis.

To sum it up, it can be said that everyone needs to know how to maintain normal and natural spinal curves. **I can undoubtedly tell you that failure to maintain the normal curves of the spine leads to a state of decreased health and a lower quality of life.**

The Functions of the Spine

The spine has several roles, the most prominent of which are protection of the spinal cord and nerves as well as movement. The spinal cord is part of the central nervous system, extends from the brain, and emerges at the height of the first lumbar vertebra. It may emerge sometimes up to one vertebra above it.

The brain is protected by the skull and the vertebrae shield and protect the spinal cord which runs through them, from external stress or stimuli, which can cause pathological damage to our bodies, such as paralysis.

The spine not only protects the spinal cord, it serves as a channel through which the nerves that emerge from it transmit messages to and from the various parts of the body. This protection allows the nerves to carry information to the brain via the spinal cord and back from the brain through the spinal cord to the body, without interference.

The spine allows the body to move in different directions, thus allowing us to perform various daily activities. The spine enables the body to bend forwards, backwards, and to bend and turn to the right and to the left.

The spine supports and assists in carrying the head, torso, chest, and upper limbs. Its stability and strength is provided by an extensive system of ligaments and muscles, all of which prevent its collapse. The thoracic vertebrae which form joints to connect with the ribs, help and participate in the breathing process.

The Importance of the Pelvis

The pelvis is a bony area that connects the spine and legs and creates a space that contains blood vessels, nerves, muscles and of course the reproductive organs, (a uterus in women and a prostate gland in men,) the urinary bladder and more. The bones that make up the pelvis form attachment points for many muscles such as the abdominal muscles, back muscles, buttocks and thigh muscles.

These muscles together with the pelvic joints, allow the pelvis freedom of movement in different directions thus affecting its position, and as a result affect the position **of the vertebrae and the discs** between each vertebrae. Two significant concepts associated with poor pelvic position which can create a negative chain reaction up to the lumbar vertebrae and discs are the forward pelvic tilt and backward pelvic tilt.

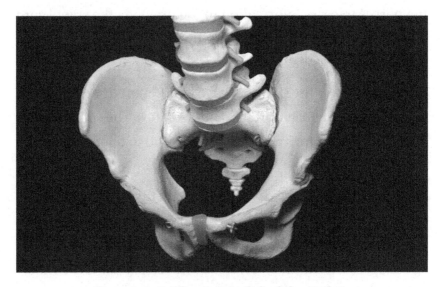

Figure 4: A Plastic Model of the Pelvis

Imagine for a moment the pelvis as a bowl of water that you hold with one hand on either side. Now tilt the front of the bowl forward and down, so the water will spill away from you. Note that the back of the bowl turns up. The pelvis can rotate forward, just like tipping the bowl forward, otherwise known as forward pelvic rotation. In reverse mode which simulates a backward rotation of the pelvis, the back of the bowl rotates down and the front part turns up, then the water will spill over you.

A backward pelvic rotation is usually related to the **straightening** of the lumbar vertebrae, which is called **Lumbar Hypolordosis,** while the **forward rotation of the pelvis usually results in the increasing and deepening of the lumbar curve,** which is called **Lumbar Hyperlordosis.**

Another impairment associated with the pelvic position is a slouched posture, in which the pelvis moves forward as a single unit. These changes in the pelvic position, some of which result from incorrect body movement and poor posture, affect the lower back, and each of them can cause problems and back pain.

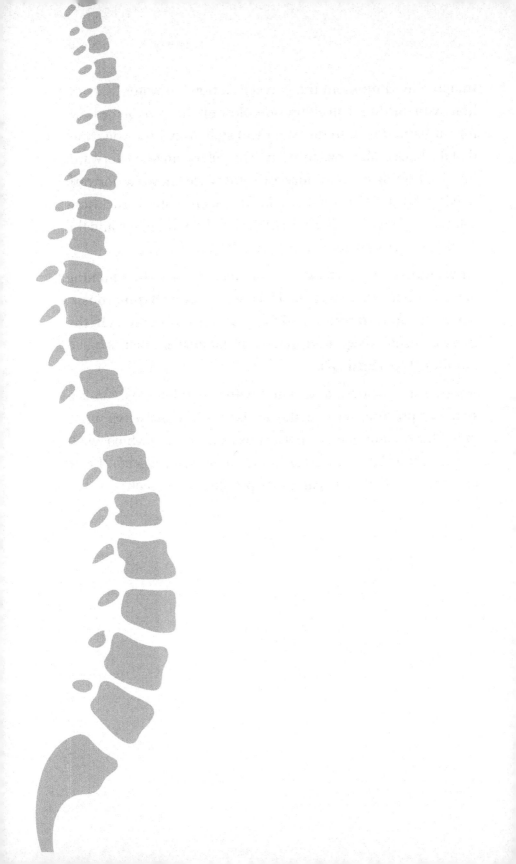

Chapter Three

The Importance of the Nervous System

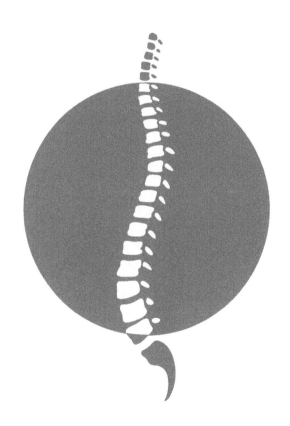

Nerves - The Most Important Wiring System You Will Ever Know!

The nervous system is the most important system in the human body. It starts from the brain, and most of it continues through the spinal cord, from which nerves emerge to all parts of the body. The proper functioning of the nerves makes every action our body does, possible. The nerves transfer the information from every cell in our body to the brain and vice versa, transferring all the information from the brain to the various body cells.

The nerves that reach muscles allow us to perform voluntary actions such as walking, jumping, lifting a hand, etc., and the nerves give commands to the muscles to contract or stretch. Nerves also control involuntary actions - actions that we have no control over - such as wound healing, heart muscle contractions, the breakdown of food in the body after swallowing, and many others. Other nerves send sensory information to the brain from a sore and painful muscle, pain in the back or a feeling of numbness in the fingers, and they are the ones that exit the brain and control the mechanism of recovery from pain.

These are only partial functions of the nerves in our bodies, and their importance and the way they operate play a significant role in our daily functioning. The skull protects the brain and the vertebrae protect the spinal cord and nerves which emerge from it.

Is it possible that the vertebrae cannot protect the nerves which pass through them in the best possible way?

Do you remember Christopher Reeve, the actor who played Superman? On May 27, 1995, he fell from a horse, broke the first two cervical vertebrae and damaged the spinal cord that passes through these vertebrae. As a result, he remained paralyzed from the neck down and with many problems in other body systems, such as the respiratory system. However, what happens to millions of people who have not experienced such a traumatic event as Christopher Reeve? Is it possible that there can be pressure on the nerves that does not result in paralysis, but 'only' causes pain in the back, neck, limbs as well as many other complaints?

To answer the question, I will give you an example from the field of agriculture. Try to imagine a garden hose which carries water to plants and trees. Try to think about what would happen to the flow of water if the inner part of the hose began to fill with rust. The speed and flow of water would most likely change accordingly, right? Meaning that the plants and trees would not receive the same amount or frequency of water and this might perhaps affect their growth and development. Now, let us say that you press lightly with your feet on the hose. The diameter of the hose will probably decrease, and there will again be a difference in the speed and flow of water. This will be reflected in a change in the way water is supplied to the plants. This may affect their growth and functioning.

Similarly, like the water in the hose, the nerves that pass through the spinal canal can be irritated and compressed, **and then their effect on the organ they are innervating (supplies with nerves) will be impaired.**

Nerves can be compressed due to several things. One is **movement of the vertebrae from their natural position**, thereby exerting pressure on the nerves. Another are **degenerative** changes in the vertebral joints and thickening of ligaments within the spinal canal (similar to rust in the pipe) which can also cause nerve pressure. If the **disc** protrudes or is displaced (slipped disc), this can cause nerve pressure (similar to the pressure applied by the foot on the hose) as well. The common denominator is pressure on a nerve or number of nerves, which can cause great suffering and significant changes to the quality of life.

In many cases, people suffer from pressure on the spinal nerves and are not aware of this phenomenon at all **due to the absence of pain** in places which the nerve innervates. **However, the damage can still occur in situations where a person does not yet suffer from any pain!** Therefore, each person should go for a periodical spinal examination.

In broad terms, the nerves that emerge from the cervical vertebrae affect the head, face, front and back of the neck, and, of course, the hands. The nerves that emerge from the thoracic vertebrae affect the internal organs in the chest and abdomen such as the heart, lungs, stomach, kidneys and intestines. The nerves that emerge from the lumbar vertebrae and the sacrum reach the organs in the lower abdomen such as the genitals, urinary bladder, bowels and, of course, the buttocks and legs. **Again, any disturbance, compression, or irritation of the nerves emerging from the spinal cord through the vertebrae will cause changes in the region that the nerves affect.**

These neurological disturbances cause our body to function inefficiently and inappropriately.

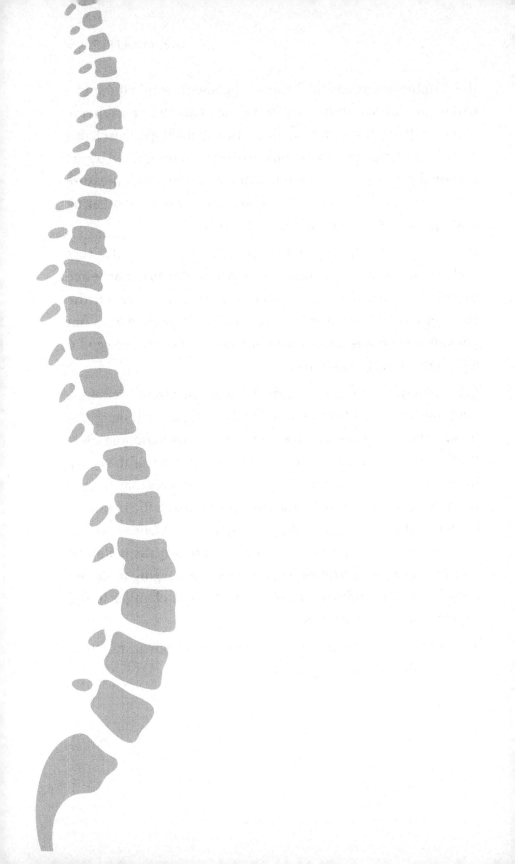

Chapter Four

Should Problems Start, Consult your Physician

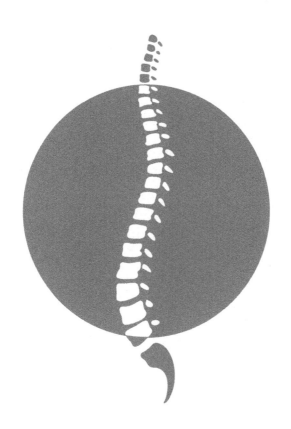

Getting to the Root of the Problem: Reasons and Problems that Cause Neck, Back and Spinal Pain

Now that we understand how our body works and the tremendous importance of the nerves which emerge from the spinal column in relation to our body systems, we will try to take a closer look at the back and neck themselves. We will try to understand what problems can arise, and what the main reasons are that can cause problems in the neck, middle back, lower back and pelvis.

There are numerous causes of pain and problems in the neck, back and spine. Pain may be due to issues in the muscles, ligaments, tendons, discs, nerves, vertebrae and pelvic bones. Trauma after a fall, a wound or an injury can cause damage to each of the above anatomical structures. Complications associated with blood vessels, inflammatory, infectious, congenital and malignancies can also cause damage to the back and great suffering to the person. Improper posture during sitting, standing, lying down, and lifting objects can cause back and neck pain as well.

Common back and spine problems that can cause great pain and frustration include:

Vertebrae

The vertebrae can move out of place: forward, backward, sideways to the right and left, and even rotate right or left. A number of vertebrae can also change their natural position, thus increasing the likelihood of pain. This, for example, can be seen in people who suffer from a hunchback (kyphosis) in which the vertebrae bend forward and downward, or in scoliosis, in which they bend and rotate sideward. A straightening of the lumbar and cervical vertebrae is quite common. When the vertebrae move out of their proper place, they press on the adjacent nerves thereby causing severe pain.

Joints

The joints of the vertebrae can degenerate and move inadequately, resulting in pain. Excessive flexibility in joints can undermine joint stability and cause pain. The joints of the vertebrae can thicken, grow, touch the nerves nearby and cause great suffering. See Figure 5 below.

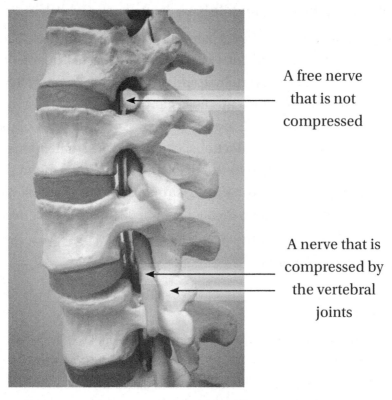

A free nerve that is not compressed

A nerve that is compressed by the vertebral joints

Figure 5: A side view of a plastic model demonstrating a number of lumbar vertebrae

Muscles

Muscles may be too short or too long, thus not allowing optimal movement in the area. Weak or contracted muscles can also cause pain.

Ligaments

The ligaments of the spine and pelvis can stretch or shorten and cause pain and restricted movement. Ligaments located inside the spinal canal can thicken and press on the nearby nerves.

Discs

The disc can degenerate and become thinner, causing the vertebrae to get closer to each other. The disc can protrude or herniate, causing local pain or even nerve pressure, refer pain to the hand or leg, and even radiate to both hands and or both legs. Any damage to the disc adversely affects the functioning of the entire area next to it. See Figure 6 below.

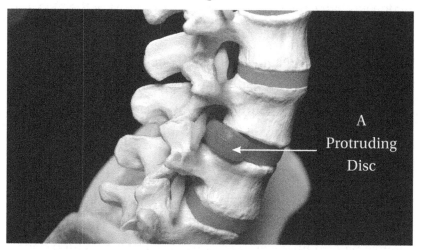

A Protruding Disc

Figure 6: A plastic model of a protruding disc

Irritated or Compressed Nerves

The nerve can be compressed by various anatomical structures such as a disc, the vertebral joints, thickening ligaments in the vertebrae, and various tumors. A very sharp pain and feelings like paresthesia (numbness), burning, 'shooting pains' in the back or limbs, weakness and other unpleasant feelings may follow.

Internal Organ Problems

Heart, kidney, intestine and liver problems can, for example, radiate pain to different areas of the back.

Other factors that can cause problems and pain are obesity, prolonged sitting at work, and various psychological factors such as pressure, stress, depression and poor posture. Sometimes back pain arises due to problems in other areas of the body, for example, flat feet (fallen arches), one shorter leg, knee, hip, shoulder, and pelvic issues. Poor vision in one eye or weak hearing in one ear can cause asymmetrical movements of the neck too, and later result in pain.

As mentioned, the causes of back, neck and spinal pain are numerous. The above list is only a partial one, so it is highly recommended to be examined by professionals.

The Suffering Engineer - David's Story

David had worked for many years as a city engineer for several authorities. A month before he showed up for treatment, he felt intense pain in his lower back and right leg. The pain relievers and Voltaren injections he received for two weeks prior to his appointment with me did not help him. A CT (Computed Tomography) scan revealed three herniated discs in his lower back.

David had received help from me in the past with cervical vertebra problems he had suffered from for years, but this was more painful and he came back to me for treatment.

David later informed me that following several treatments with me, he felt great relief and he was able to enjoy life once again. He said that he regretted suffering through two weeks of agony before contacting me, and added that if he had seen me earlier, he would have saved himself a great deal of suffering.

●●●

What is My Spine Trying to Tell Me? Symptoms that May Occur Due to Spinal Problems

Most people do not go for regular checkups and only go to a doctor if something happens to them. Pain is the most common complaint of people seeking medical help. The most common areas of pain due to spinal problems are the neck and lower back, followed by pain in the middle of the back and between the shoulder blades. Pain may be experienced while sitting, standing up, lying down, turning around in bed, getting up in the morning, or from coughing, and can make life in general very difficult. Many people suffer from pain due to many years of neglect, and only the intensification of the pain causes them to seek medical help.

I suggest that you do not make the mistake that many tend to make. People ignore low or intermittent pain, do not get examined, and in some cases the increase in pain levels causes them to suffer much more - which makes it more difficult to help them due to their new acute condition.

Many patients who come to my clinic complain that their pain began in the lower back and that after a few days or a week, it was accompanied by pain along the entire length of the leg. The symptoms included, for example, paresthesia, a tingling pain, a stabbing pain, 'shooting pains', heat or a burning sensation, sometimes accompanied by weakness of the leg. Most of them admit that failing to seek immediate help was a significant mistake, and now, when their problem is more complex, they understand that they will have to undergo many more expensive treatment sessions with less chance of recovery because their bodies may have irreversible damage.

A problem in the neck can cause similar symptoms such as tingling, 'shooting pains' and pain in the shoulder, arm, forearm, palm and fingers, and some might even have difficulty with simple motor functions such as buttoning a shirt or gripping lightweight objects such as a fork and plate.

Some of my patients tell me that the pain they experienced in the neck or lower back diminished, but was **replaced** by increased symptoms in the hands or legs. This indicates a **deterioration** in health which requires rapid medical assistance in order to provide a quick response to the patient's problem.

Problems in the neck, back, and spine can lead to pain in other areas of the body, such as chest pain, shoulder or knee pain, cramps, pain in leg muscles and headaches. Additional complaints by the patient can include respiratory discomfort, weakness in the limbs, dizziness, frequent urination, and many other complaints.

These are just a number of examples of problems that I have chosen to share with you, problems that most people don't realize may originate from the spine.

Headaches

Many people suffer from headaches and try to get rid of them in a variety of ways. Because headaches are very common, many people think that headaches are an integral part of their lives. But they are wrong!

Some suffer from chronic headaches and migraines for many years. Drug therapy or any other conservative treatment does not always solve the problem. In my experience, chiropractic care can help with this problem.

There are many reasons for headaches, but a common cause that many people are not aware of is improper spinal function, especially of the neck vertebrae, the upper thoracic vertebrae, and the anatomical structures associated with them.

When spinal vertebrae move from their position (move within the neck) or do not move normally (a decrease in the range of movement of the neck in one or more directions), pressure may occur on the nerves and blood vessels, which is interpreted as a headache.

Degenerative changes such as small protuberances (bony overgrowth) from the vertebrae, a herniated disc in the neck or thickening of the joints of the cervical vertebrae, can narrow the intervertebral canal through which the nerve passes and cause irritation to the nerve, leading to symptoms such as neck and head pain.

It is important to remember that the nerves that emerge from the upper cervical vertebrae reach the head area, and if irritated or compressed, they may cause headaches and may even cause pain in the eye.

Prolonged sitting in front of a computer, road accidents, poor posture, etc., can cause chronic or acute stretching of the neck muscles that connect to the occiput (back bone of the skull), resulting in neck pain and headaches.

Degenerative changes in the joints of the cervical vertebrae can cause pressure on the vertebral artery that passes through the cervical vertebrae and cause chronic headaches.

Chiropractic treatment performed after a comprehensive examination can achieve many benefits. Among other things, these treatments can release the 'fixed' vertebrae or the vertebrae that is not moving optimally, thereby reducing pressure off the blood vessels, muscles and nerves in the neck area.

Successful treatment allows proper functioning of the nervous system and delays the pace of joint degeneration.

"My Smile Returned" – Dan's Story

Dan, a man in his fifties, showed up at my clinic on the recommendation of a relative who I had previously treated. He complained of pain in the cervical spine area, from which he had been suffering for several years. He had difficulty in performing basic neck movements, a hard time lifting his hands and carrying objects, pains in his arms and shoulders, headaches and dizziness.

A magnetic resonance imaging scan (MRI) of the neck showed disc protrusions from the fourth to the seventh cervical vertebra with nerve pressure, degenerative changes in the vertebral joints and pressure on the spinal cord.

Before he had arrived at my clinic, Dan had undergone a year of a variety of treatments, but to no avail. During the ten treatments that Dan underwent at my clinic, he recorded that his smile had 'returned', his neck pain was reduced, the headaches were better, and his ability to move his neck had improved greatly.

●●●

Respiratory Discomfort – Rachel's Story

Rachel, a woman of about 50, came to me with complaints of pain in her neck, shoulder blade, and upper back. She told me that for years, she had been sitting with her head bent forward in front of the computer in her office, but lately the pains had increased. She said that she even felt respiratory discomfort, which required her to occasionally use an inhaler. She denied any injury in the area, and underwent various cardiac tests that found nothing.

When I examined her, I immediately saw that her head tilted forward in comparison to her upper body, her shoulders rotated inward with restricted movement in the upper thoracic vertebrae, resulting in noticeable stiffness. The muscles between the shoulder blades and the spine were also very sensitive to touch.

I decided to combine several types of treatment to help her: stretching the chest muscles, strengthening the muscles in the neck and the shoulder blades, and different techniques of moving the fixed vertebrae (mobilization and manipulations). Rachel's improvement was rapid and included a significant reduction of pain, dramatic relief of breathing, and no further need of an inhaler. Rachel has since been in periodic preventive care to prevent the return of these problems and to minimize the probability of new problems as much as possible.

● ● ●

Lost Money - Ethan's Story

Have you ever been confused when counting coins? Did you ever lose bills without realizing it? Maybe not, but if so, probably very rarely. But there are people who do lose money quite frequently.

Ethan showed up at my clinic with pains in his neck and right hand. He told me that he had numbness or decreased sensation in the fingers of his right hand. In a cervical X-ray, I could see degenerative changes in the lower cervical vertebrae, as well as **narrowing** of the intervertebral canals through which the nerves pass into the hands.

He reported that he had complained about this for a long time. An examination showed that the lower cervical vertebrae were responsible for the poor sensation in his fingers, since there was pressure on the nerves that emerge from these vertebrae which causes numbness in the fingers and impaired sensation. I explained to him that due to the chronic severity of his problem, he needed a series of treatments, which I performed.

At the end of the treatment, he took out his wallet, paid me and left. A few minutes later, I noticed that two hundred-dollar bills were on the floor. The problem in the cervical vertebrae had caused him to lose sensation in his fingers, and the bills had fallen from his hands without him realizing.

I called him and he confirmed that this kind of situation did happen to him from time to time. The treatments he received improved the impaired sensation in his fingers and reduced his neck pain. When he came back to the clinic, I gave him back his money, and that evening he took his wife to a fancy restaurant.

● ●●

This phenomenon of numbness in the fingers is very common. In some cases this is due to diabetes, and sometimes it is due to irritation of the nerves emerging from the lower cervical vertebrae. The irritation of these nerves can also cause weakness in various places along the hand.

It is not worth waiting for pain to appear, and only then to take care of the body.

Pain is the last symptom that appears.

The damage occurs before the onset of pain. I strongly recommend that you have your back examined today to avoid problems tomorrow.

●●●

Problems in the Left Leg – Sharon's Story

After more than twenty years of helping thousands of patients, I know that the most common complaint is lower back pain that affects the leg - a complaint that actually disrupts the patient's quality of life and causes great suffering. Sharon is one of many who came to me with a complaint about lower back pain and pain in her left external lower leg, with numbness in her little toe on the left foot.

I got the impression that Sharon was very tired, and I immediately suspected that because of her pain, she could not sleep well at night. "Do you suffer from pain during the night?" I asked. She replied affirmatively that her leg mainly bothered her at night and that twice a week she even suffered cramps in her left calf, which made her jump out of bed.

I understood that most of Sharon's complaints stemmed from the various symptoms she had with her leg, which she shared with me in great detail, and that her back bothered her less at this stage. Sharon wanted to know if there was a specific treatment for her leg in order to alleviate her suffering. Although I explained to Sharon that it was imperative to first examine the CT images of her back, she still insisted that the problem was her leg, not her back.

After an in-depth study of the images, I made it clear to her that a lumbar disc herniation at L5-S1 was pressing on the root of the nerve, on the left side, and gently pushing it. This caused the symptoms she felt in her leg. Therefore, if we could manage to rehabilitate the problematic area of her lower back, we would see an improvement in her leg.

Based on years of experience with other patients who experienced symptoms similar to hers, I explained to Sharon that a series of intensive **back** treatments could speed up the recovery process of her leg.

During the course of treatment, Sharon reported that the cramps she suffered at night began to disappear and she felt a significant decrease in pain in her leg and partial return of sensation in the small toe.

Doctor, Do I Have a Back Problem?

When you visit your doctor, try telling him the most important information about your complaint, problem, or pain. It is recommended to explain exactly when and how the pain began, the type of pain, what eases or intensifies the pain, its location and severity. Your doctor will perform a physical examination and will be able to perform various, more specific spinal tests such as a static and dynamic assessment of your vertebrae, a posture examination, specific muscle tests, etc.

If necessary, the doctor will refer you to additional doctors for further opinions, further tests, or to speed up the treatment. Your doctor may need to refer you for spinal X-rays or even advanced imaging tests such as Computed Tomography (CT), Magnetic Resonance Imaging (MRI), bone scan and other tests.

Additionally, your doctor may refer you for various blood tests so that he can treat you more specifically later on.

After this process, your doctor will give you a diagnosis and recommend the best treatment options available for your condition.

I Have a Back Problem, What Should I Do?

Once the doctor has examined you and used various tests to find your problem, you will receive an explanation on what treatment options are available to help you. In most cases, a combination of treatments at the doctor's clinic, along with various instructions that the doctor will ask you to carry out in your own time, are the therapeutic options that can help you and accelerate your recovery. I recommend that you contact a doctor you know and trust so that he can offer you the best advice on how to resolve your problem.

I would like to also recommend two methods of action. The first one is advice and treatment by the attending physician, and the other is concurrent maintenance of correct posture and movement of your body, as will be explained in the book later on. I believe that following these methods will prevent irreversible damage to your body and, in addition, improve the quality of your life.

I often hear from veteran patients that they continue to follow my recommendations, perform specific back exercises and that they work on their back and neck on a daily basis. They are pleased that the difficult and acute situation they had initially felt is now a thing of the past and they believe that by implementing my guidelines, they will avoid future spinal problems.

Back pain is one of the most common complaints of people in the health field. The scope of the phenomenon is so widespread that it seems that every person will suffer from it at least once in his life. The saying goes that the world's population is divided into two, those who have back pain and those who will have back pain.

Back pain is the cause of much suffering to millions of people worldwide and impairs their quality of life. Back pain is also one of the main reasons for taking sick days from work, and it can even lead to an inability to work.

Many billions of dollars are wasted every year because of the financial consequences of back pain. This is reflected in payments for medical examinations, counseling, and various treatments, loss of work productivity for employers, and financial payments to people due to temporary or permanent back pain.

After many years of helping numerous people, I want to ensure you that **there is light at the end of the tunnel,** and that back pain can be improved both in chronic and acute situations.

If you have already tried a certain method of treatment for your specific problem, and have experienced minor progress, you should know that there are many other treatments available and even alternative therapies may help you. **So do not despair!**

When to Seek Urgent Medical Help?

There are certain situations in which we should immediately contact and consult with a doctor and be treated in the fastest and most effective manner:

- **Weight loss or fever** - the appearance of back pain accompanied by a prolonged and involuntary decrease in weight or body temperature, requires immediate investigation.

- **Trauma** - acute pain anywhere in the spine and back as a result of trauma such as a car accident or falling on your back requires immediate medical treatment.

- **Neurology** - neurological exacerbation or the sudden onset of a neurological problem such as significant weakness in the limbs, foot drop, sudden speech impairment, walking instability, and lack of bladder or bowel control are examples in which a person should seek urgent medical assistance.

- **Incontinence** - the spinal cord ends either at thoracic vertebra 12 or at the first lumbar vertebrae. A relatively rare phenomenon may occur when pressure on the roots of the nerves that emerge below the end of the spinal cord, inside the spinal canal, induce pressure and cause signs and symptoms of lack of voluntary control over the bowels and urinary bladder, severe weakness of the legs and numbness in the anus and pelvis. These symptoms require urgent medical intervention.

In all of these situations, you should consult a physician as soon as possible to avoid irreversible damage.

Having read how to identify back, neck, and spinal problems, I guess you would like to read on, and learn how to reduce aches and pains. Continue reading to receive good and beneficial advice!

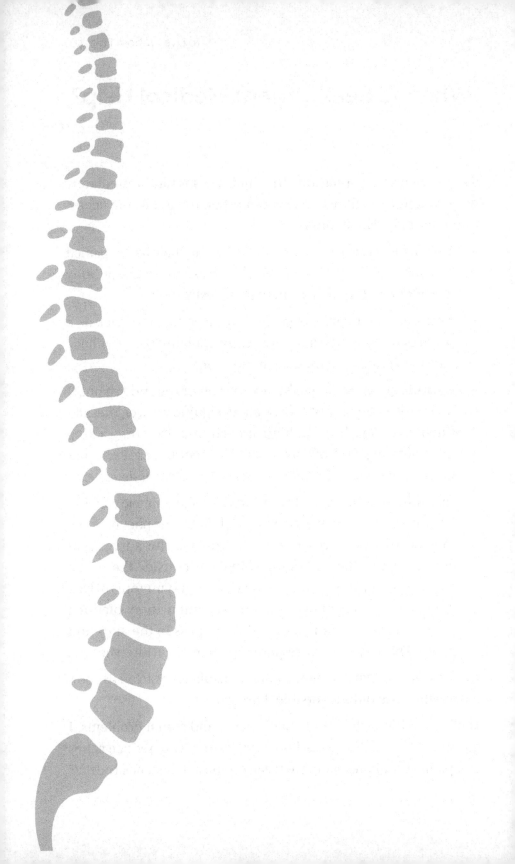

Chapter Five
Solutions Revealed

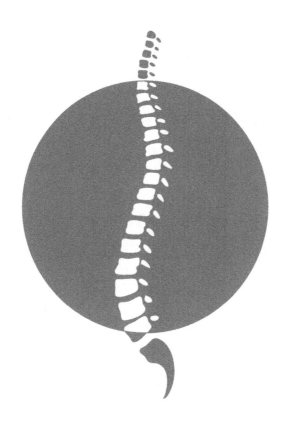

Correct Posture

The Importance of Learning Correct Posture to Prevent Spinal Impairments

Many back problems occur as a result of incorrect posture. The way we sit, stand, lie down, bend, move objects and move around in general is very important to prevent damage to our spine and even alleviate existing problems. Incorrect posture may result in improper transition of weight to various parts of the body and can cause abnormal functioning of the body.

Incorrect posture causes the various body systems and internal organs to operate sub-optimally and expend unnecessary energy and effort. Think, for example, of people who constantly bend their head, shoulders and body. This will compress their chests and adversely affect their breathing. Is it possible that the same person will suffer from neck pain, shoulder blade aches, pain in the shoulders, and perhaps frequent headaches as a result of poor posture? The answer is **of course!**

Our posture depends on the genetics we receive from our parents and the habits we acquire during our lives. The difference between the sexes which is expressed, among other things, by the structure of the body, e.g. the pelvis, difference in muscular mass, and in the density and strength of the bones, are all important components of our posture. Posture also varies according to age as over the years, there are various degenerative spinal changes and the natural spinal curves have a tendency to decrease. Emotional elements such as sadness, depression, lack of social acceptance, along with low self-esteem, can result in a slumped and bent posture that will lead to various structural and functional problems in the spine and back. Of course, our work environment also has great impact on our posture, and it is vital that each and every one of us receives professional guidance on this important subject.

During my many years of working with patients, I have noticed that a high percentage of them **do not apply** the principles of proper posture. So, many of them suffer from neck and back problems, and many others will suffer from them in the future. One of the major problems is that old habits die hard! However, it is always better to try to change to good habits, no matter what your age. This requires knowledge, patience and practice in order to improve general body behavior.

Of course, it is better to learn and be educated about correct posture and good back health from an early age. One of my goals is to provide children and youth with theoretical and practical knowledge of optimal body behavior in order to save them significant problems in the future. One of the main ways to address this need is via lectures which I give to students and to the public, providing information and many valuable tips on the subject.

After my compulsory military service, I decided to attend the Wingate College, in Israel, where I studied physical education with the intention of becoming a Physical Education teacher. At Wingate, my B.A. studies included specializing in the promotion of correct posture and preventative exercises. As part of my studies, I examined elementary school children for spinal column impairments, such as scoliosis, kyphosis (humpback), a too-straight back, hyperlordosis (excessive inward lumbar curve), and other problems. After determining the diagnosis, the therapeutic stage began. This included, among other things, shortening and lengthening muscles, strengthening specific muscles, posture exercises tailored to address specific back issues, etc.

When I was in elementary school, I remember that the school nurse would conduct periodic posture examinations on all students. I do not think that these tests are conducted in schools today, and that is a shame. Our responsibility is to make this knowledge accessible to everyone we know - children and adults - so that they may enjoy a better quality of life no matter their age.

Six Ways to Detect Spinal Impairments with a Posture Test

It is important to adopt correct postural habits for as many hours during the day as possible. These habits should be applied in static situations, while sitting or standing and in motional activities such as walking and changing positions, for example getting out of bed or getting into a vehicle.

Here are some ways to test your personal posture:

1. **Examination by a doctor or a professional.** It is recommended that each and every one of us to be examined by a professional (orthopedist, chiropractor, Alexander method expert, etc.) who will analyze our posture during movement and at rest, whether at home or at work. Impairments discovered during posture examination may indicate spinal and back problems, and if you work to correct them, you can save problems, pain and suffering, and particularly in your spine. In addition, you will receive a great deal of information during this type of examination that will help solve your spinal problems, should you have any.

2. **Environmental feedback**. Take a few moments and try to think if you have ever been told that you sit with a bent back and need to sit straighter. Have you ever been told by family or friends that your posture is incorrect? If so, you should think about these comments and consult a professional.

3. **Looking at photos and personal videos**. I recommend you review photos and videos of yourself on your computer, phone,

or in photo albums. Look at yourself. Do you sit or stand with a straight or bent back? Does your head lean forward compared with the rest of your body? Are you leaning to one side? Do you have a hump in the middle of your back or upper torso?

This is a great way to gather information about yourself. Try to see if there are consistent signs that you see in multiple images, as this may become a steady pattern.

4. **A self-symmetry test in front of the mirror**. Stand in front of a full size mirror that allows you to see your whole body. Look at yourself from your head down to your feet. Study each part of your body for 10 seconds to check your posture. The goal is to see if there are any symmetrical differences between the right side and the left side.

Start from your head: Is it in the middle or leaning to one side? Are your ears the same height? Move on to your shoulders: Are they the same height or is one higher than the other? Now look at the distance between the elbows on the inside of your arms in comparison to your ribs. Compare the distance between the right side of your body and your left side.

Next, slide your hands from the ribs down your torso, until you feel the pelvic bones. Place your hands on the pelvic bones in a stable position for a few seconds, and again compare the height of your pelvis between the right and left sides.

Bring your hands back to your sides. Try to feel whether you divide your weight equally on your feet or whether you have a problem with your back or one leg that causes uneven weight loads to your feet. Try to determine whether you stand on your entire foot or tend to stand on the inside or outside edge of the foot? Keep looking down at your legs and feet.

Are your knees the same height? Is one knee slightly bent in relation to the other?

Finally, look at your feet. Do they point outwards? Inwards? Or are they parallel to each other and open out slightly (optimal mode)?

It is advisable to make a record of the signs you have discovered during your examination and to consult with a professional who can verify or deny the findings and provide medical response as necessary and as soon as possible. Findings in this examination can indicate back and spinal impairments even if you are not suffering from back pain at present. Signs detected in this examination can also indicate additional impairments not caused by the spine, but which have an effect on the back and spine.

5. **Check for symmetry and possible impairments with the help of another person in front of the mirror.** You can ask a friend or relative to perform an additional test and you can then exchange notes. If someone else examines you, they can stand behind you and ask you to bend forward with an arched back. They can then look at your back and see if there is a hump or arch that appears on one side which does not appear on the other side, which frequently indicates scoliosis. Also, that person can observe as you bend your own back right and left while standing, and see whether the range of motion is the same on each side.

6. **Side-view mirror inspection**. Now switch to a side-view inspection. Here too, a self-examination is not accurate enough, and you should consult a professional. Even so, such an examination will provide you with some preliminary information about your posture. In this examination, you will

try to see whether your back maintains the natural curves of the spine or not, and whether there are areas or organs that have moved from their optimal place.

First, look at your whole body. Is it relatively straight or is there a tendency to lean forward? Now keep looking at your body, starting with your head, and gradually look down. Are your head and neck in line with your upper torso or are they leaning forward and hunched? Does the ear and shoulder create an imaginary **vertical** line between the two (normal), or does your ear look more forward in comparison to your shoulder? Go to the mid-back area, between the shoulder blades. Is it protruding backwards too much? A little conspicuous? Alternatively, is it not noticeable at all? Remember, there should be a slight arch of the back in this area.

Continue down and look at your abdomen. Is it protruding forward and falling, which can adversely affect the lower back, or is it flat and slightly collected inward? Look at your buttocks. Are they very prominent? This could increase the risk of back pain.

Try looking at your lower back. Do you notice a lumbar depression? Is it very noticeable or is there no depression at all, and you think the vertebrae have straightened? Just as a reminder, there should be a lumbar depression. Straightening of the vertebrae or too much depression is not an optimal back condition.

Finally, look at your knees down to your ankles. Are your knees bent, which can indicate a backward pelvic rotation (as explained in chapter two)? Are they locked and create a relative vertical line between the hip and the thigh? Alternatively, is the knee in a state of hyperextension, which can cause the pelvis to tilt forward and even affect the position of the lower back vertebrae?

In conclusion, this posture test can give you some initial and potentially extensive information about how your posture affects your body in general. Finding possible impairments in this test can indicate changes in your back and spine that require further investigation to prevent further problems in your body.

Potential Damage Due to the Incorrect Position of the Head and Neck

One of the most common posture dysfunctions is related to the position of the neck and head. During our lives, we spend too many hours in activities that cause the head and neck to bend and move forward, therefore the chance of damage to our neck increases. See Figure 7 below. Actions that cause the head to bend forward, such as the use of cell phones while standing or sitting, using the computer at home and at work, lying on the back and using several pillows to support the head - some examples of this common phenomenon - may adversely affect our health. In addition, many professionals, e.g., secretaries, alternative medicine therapists who practice reflexology, masseurs, pedicurists and manicurists, all hold their neck and head in unnatural positions for a length of time which can lead to damage.

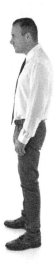

Figure 7: Incorrect Standing Posture

Lack of awareness of proper posture, laziness, accidents and wear as a result of age also exacerbate the phenomenon of bending the head forward.

Optimal posture can be seen when looking at a person from a side view; the shoulder and the ear are in a vertical line. See figure 8 below.

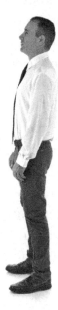

Figure 8: Correct Standing Posture

When the head and neck move forward, we do not see a vertical line and the ear will be forward in comparison to the shoulder. This condition is not healthy for the neck and shoulder blades because the mechanical stress on the anatomical structures in the neck increases which can cause serious functional problems later on.

This poor posture, in which the forward position of the head causes the neck and shoulder muscles to stretch and the cervical vertebrae to move forward, requires more effort to be applied in order to prevent the head from falling forwards. As the head moves further forward, the distance between the ear and the shoulder increases, and the weight load on anatomical structures in the neck such as muscles, ligaments and discs increases, thereby increasing the risk of damage.

In this forward-tilted head posture, the chances of seeing degenerative changes in the vertebrae and discs increases, and later disc problems may occur, such as disc protrusion or disc herniation. Common symptoms are headaches, neck and shoulder pain, movement restrictions in the neck and shoulders, and even various complaints in the upper limbs as a result of pressure on the nerves which emerge out of the lower cervical vertebrae.

Some people with this condition complain of a strange feeling in the hands, especially a numbness in their palms and fingers while others complain about a burning sensation or weakness in the hand.

It is important to remember that the nerves coming from the lower cervical vertebrae and upper chest vertebrae also reach the heart and lungs.

Sometimes forward tilting of the cervical and thoracic vertebrae, accompanied by a forward rotation of the shoulders and a shortening of the chest muscles, cause a slight constriction of the chest. This, combined with the same possible pressure on the nerves, may cause changes in the functioning of the heart and lung system, to occur.

Therefore, we must be aware of correct posture and the severe consequences that poor posture can lead to, and make an effort to maintain proper posture where the ear and shoulder form a vertical imaginary line.

Possible Damages Caused by Prolonged Bending of the Middle Back

One of the significant impairments seen in the back is the excessive bending and arching of the middle of the back and the area between the shoulder blades. This is due to the fact that too much time is spent during the day in a state of bending of the middle of the back. This impairment of bending and arching is very common and can cause health damage and significantly harm our quality of life. See Figure 9 below.

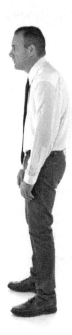

Figure 9: Excessive bending of the middle back and the area between the shoulder blades

Normally, in a side view of the dorsal spine, the part between the neck and the lower back, should be slightly arched. As a result of various causes, the middle of the back bends excessively and causes the vertebrae to bend and compress, more so in the front, and the back muscles to lengthen and stretch, thus increasing the chances of back pain. In a minor number of cases, the reason for this is congenital and is manifested in hyperkyphosis, usually due to a defect in the vertebrae, or sometimes due to various diseases.

In most cases, the middle of the back is bent because of bad habits. Prolonged sitting in front of a computer over many years, laziness and lack of postural awareness causing a slumped sitting position, and sitting too much in general, are the most common causes of a bend in the middle of the back. Sometimes a low self-image or body image, shyness, prolonged depression, lack of coming to terms with body shape and/or weight, or social rejection may result in a bending of the upper back and shoulder blades. Other causes, such as aging of the spine, osteoporosis, or shoulder and lower back problems, can adversely affect the middle of the back and cause it to bend as well.

This bending of the thoracic vertebrae can cause confined and restricted movement of the back in different directions, poor movement of the joints of the vertebrae, lengthening and weakening of the back muscles, all resulting in back pain. In this situation, the shoulder blades and shoulders change their optimal position by bending forward, thus increasing the likelihood of increased functional problems, pain in the hands, shoulder blades and shoulders. Numbness and 'shooting pains' may even be felt in the hands.

Because the dorsal vertebrae in the middle of the back bend and change their position, chain reactions are created that reach the neck and lower back, and pain may appear in these areas as well. In addition, there may be additional symptoms such as headaches and pelvic pain.

The dorsal vertebrae in this region are attached to the ribs, and their chronic bending also cause the ribs to bend down, reducing movement of the chest and affecting respiratory function.

Prolonged and chronic bending of the vertebrae causes compression of the internal organs such as the heart, lungs and liver, along with degenerative changes in the vertebrae. This causes increased stress on the nerves that supply these organs, and leads to **abnormal functioning of these organs**, even if there is no pain! This poor posture, in addition to being unattractive, entails significant damage to our health and requires us to work to reduce its occurrence in order to improve our quality of life.

The solution is possible only after we have determined the main factor of poor posture. Some therapeutic options of this problem include increasing correct posture awareness; reducing sitting time and understanding correct sitting positions; exercises to stretch the chest muscles; strengthening muscles of the back, the neck and shoulder blades; correct and controlled sports activity to improve lung function; active and passive activation of dorsal spine vertebrae; and maintaining normal movement of the shoulders. All this can be done, of course, after seeking medical consultation on the subject.

My Grandfather's Posture at the Age of 100!

My grandfather, Shmuel Odrozhinsky, was born in 1911 in a small village two kilometers from the town of Janow, Poland. When he was young, he used to walk this distance daily from his home to school and back. As an adult, he made his living as a tailor. In pictures from his youth, he appears upright and it is clear that he had correct posture.

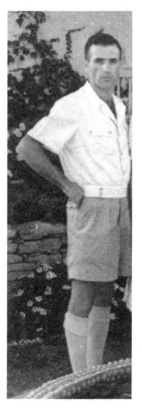

Photo of my Grandfather Samuel in his Youth

In 1939, he set off on his journey to the Land of Israel, a journey in which he experienced many hardships, since he immigrated to Israel illegally. For three months he stayed at sea, during which time he and the other passengers were forced to abandon their ship "Chapo" when it ran aground and boarded a different ship named "Katina". At the end of this journey, the British arrested him with his friends; they were held in detention for some time before finally being released.

Grandfather lived in Haifa's Neve Sha'anan neighborhood, in a fourth floor apartment without an elevator. Many times during the day, he would go up and down all those steps in addition to walking several kilometers a day at a brisk pace.

As I watched him over the years, through the eyes of an expert on posture and spine, I realized that he maintained two functional principles important for longevity and good quality of life. One is cardiovascular endurance, and the other is erect posture. Walking up and down stairs a number of times per day, as well as taking daily walks, allows the muscles of the legs to become stronger, thus reducing stresses that could reach and damage the vertebrae and discs. In addition, these actions enabled the heart to function more efficiently and to normalize blood flow to the various parts of the body. Correct posture, such as my grandfather's, not bent or slumped, allows better functional activity of the various organs of the body, especially the back.

Although my grandfather had lost most of his family in the Holocaust, and his daughter who died at the age of thirty-four, he was blessed with strong mental health and excellent physical health. The whole family was really surprised when, after the age of 100, he started to fail physically. We thought he would live for many more years.

The local municipality where he lived, in cooperation with the National Insurance Institute, holds an annual ceremony for "young" pensioners who reach the age of **100**. The picture below shows my grandfather, my daughter Yuval and me, photographed after the ceremony. Here, too, his erect posture can clearly be seen. It was a proud moment for us, attending the ceremony.

A few months later, towards the end of 2011, my grandfather and I stayed in a hotel at the Dead Sea for three days. He went into the hot tub, enjoyed the salt pools and in the evenings we went for walks outside. My grandfather did not need any walking aids nor did he experience any pain during the trip and it is an experience that I will never forget.

I strongly advise everyone to receive medical consultation on proper posture, as it can contribute to a better quality of life and longevity.

Grandfather died in 2013.

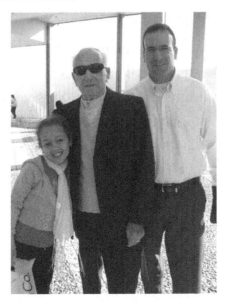

Photo of my Grandfather, aged 100 after the Ceremony.

The Natural Curves of My Spine are Almost Unnoticeable. Is that Good?

We are often told, "Keep your back straight." However, is a straight back good for our health? Is a straight back the key to good health?

Looking at a side view of an adult, the ideal position for proper posture is an inward curve in the cervical and lumbar areas, and an outward curve in the dorsal region (read about spinal curves in the basic concept section).

There are different situations in which the lower back vertebrae change their position and straighten, and even create a chain reaction up in the middle vertebrae, until the spine straightens as well. See Figure 10 below. This may be diagnosed by X-ray, and even by a clinical examination.

A straight back may look aesthetically more beautiful, but functionally it is not optimal. The spinal curves usually seen from a side view disappear and all you will see is a straight back. Spinal curves are important because they help minimize stress and shocks to the spinal column and the body. When the vertebrae straighten, the mechanism for absorbing the shocks is deficient and exposes the spine to injuries.

Have you ever 'missed' a step going downstairs, when your leg is straight instead of being slightly bent? The feeling is not good, and you get a sharp pain in the back. The same thing happens with a straight back: its ability to absorb shocks is reduced and even simple actions can cause acute pain.

So why does the lower back straighten? Most of us sit for many hours working in front of a computer, at home in front of the television, and during prolonged sitting in a car. When we sit, the pelvis moves down and rotates backwards, in most cases causing straightening of the lumbar vertebrae and increasing the load on the intervertebral discs. Proper posture awareness may prevent backward pelvic rotation and straightening of the vertebrae.

The pelvis can also rotate backwards because of the impact of muscles attached to it. For example, shortening of the hamstrings, located at the back of the thigh, can cause a backward rotation of the pelvis and straightening of the lumbar vertebrae. This straightening can cause a chain reaction to the spinal vertebrae above and straighten them as well.

However, extending these muscles will allow the vertebrae to return to their natural position. Degenerative changes in intervertebral discs, which result in their thinning and therefore loss of height, cause the lumbar vertebrae to move close together and straighten. In these situations, flexibility and strengthening exercises to strengthen the back muscles and create a lumbar curve may help improve the vertebral position.

To summarize, in most cases when you tell a person to straighten their back, it usually means that they are currently in a bent position and that they have to straighten up, which is a correct observation. Nevertheless, a spine that is too erect is not recommended. The best situation is to maintain the natural and existing curves of the spine.

As previously mentioned, it is always recommended to perform a professional posture examination in order to locate postural impairments, if any, as early as possible, in order to save much suffering in the future.

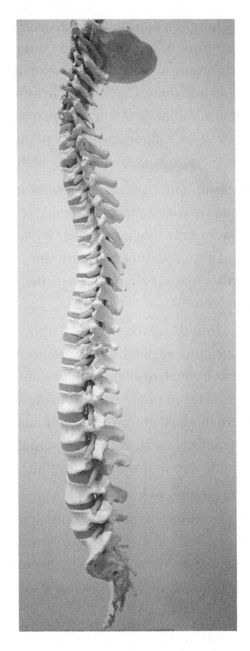

Figure 10: A side view of a plastic spine model, demonstrating reduced spinal curves. Straightening of the Spine

Learn How to Overcome an Exaggerated Lumbar Curve

There are situations in which the vertebrae in the lower back move from their natural position, causing the shock-absorbing mechanism of the vertebrae to not function optimally.

Imagine holding a flexible tube in the palm of your hand at the bottom and placed vertically on the table.

Now press lightly downward with the other hand on the top of the tube. A curve forms in the inner part of the tube. The position of the vertebrae in the lower back in their normal state is similar to the tube. However, what happens if we bend the tube even further, so that the edges are closer to each other? The curve grows. In this condition of excessive curvature, a deeper arch of the vertebrae is created - this can occur in the neck or lower back. See Figure 11 below.

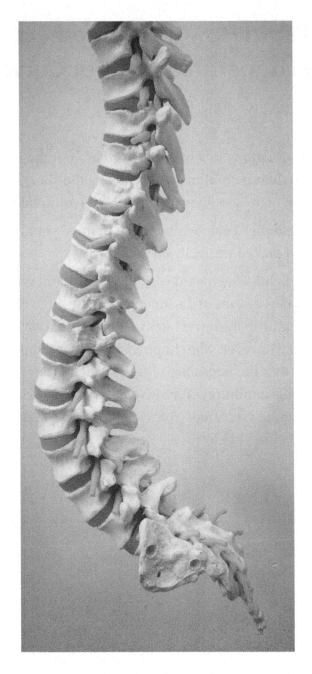

Figure 11: A plastic model of the vertebrae demonstrating an exaggerated lumbar curve.

An exaggerated lumbar curve can also begin in the fetal period as a result of changes in the position and shape of the vertebrae, and may also appear in people as a result of poor body activity. For example, excessive weight on the vertebrae as a result of weight gain during pregnancy, uncontrolled weightlifting, poor posture, or repeated backward bends such as those performed by dancers, can cause the same exaggerated arching of the lower back vertebrae.

The vertebrae in this condition are compressed and move closer to one another at the rear part creating pressure and stress, especially on the joints between the vertebrae and on the disc, which is then expressed by back pain. These pains usually occur while standing, walking, and even swimming the breaststroke.

Compression of the vertebrae also causes narrowing of the openings through which the nerves emerge and subjects them to increased pressure. Pressing of cervical nerves can cause numbness and a tingling sensation in the hands, headaches, neck pain and more. Pressure on the lower back nerves due to excessive overextension of the lumbar vertebrae can cause numbness, shooting pains and cramps in the legs, along with changes in bowel movement, frequent urination, and an effect on the genitals such as testicular pain.

Uncontrolled sport activity, as well as lack of physical activity, can cause movement of the vertebrae from their natural optimal position causing hyperextension (arching).

Weak abdominal muscles and weak hip extensor muscles at the back of the thigh and pelvis can cause the pelvis to rotate forward and result in hyperextension of the vertebrae. Similarly, muscles that are too short at the front of the pelvis and upper thigh, as well as in the lower back, will also cause a forward pelvic rotation and hyperextension of the lower back vertebrae.

People with an exaggerated lumbar curve may be identified by their posture. Usually, their abdomens protrude forward, while the buttocks protrude backwards.

How can patients with hyperlordosis symptoms get relief? The main idea is to perform actions that straighten the lumbar curve. For example, you can simultaneously bring both your knees toward your chest while laying down on your back. It is recommended to perform this exercise several times a day and to remain static in this position, with gentle movements.

Strengthening the abdominal muscles, especially the vertical abdominal muscle (rectus abdominis), is very important in this condition, as this muscle can cause backward pelvic rotation and reduce the angle of the excessive lumbar curve. There are also various stretching treatment methods , similar to the tube I mentioned at the beginning of the chapter, in which the ends of the tube are stretched and move away from each other. This action can help reduce back and neck pain and even allow the nerves to function better because less pressure is being exerted on them on their way to the organs.

As always, I recommend consulting with a professional to receive ideal therapeutic guidance.

Standing

Learn How to Reduce and Even Prevent Back Pain While Standing

Many people experience back pain when they are just standing still. This astonishes them because they do not seem to be exerting any spinal stress, so they do not understand why they have back pain. This certainly happens to people whose work involves prolonged standing, such as schoolteachers, hairdressers and store salespeople, and can even happen when you are standing in line to pay at a store. The pain can cause great frustration and can interfere with daily functioning.

The Story of Ben- the Bartender's Back Pain

Ben is a law student who works weekends as a bartender in a pub near his home. His work requires prolonged standing behind the bar, preparing drinks and serving them to the customers at the bar, and filling orders for the waitresses who serve drinks to the tables. Ben claims that his lower back pain really bothers him during his eight-hour shift and makes it difficult for him to concentrate on his work.

●●●

So why do Ben and many others suffer pain while standing? When standing for a long time in one spot, the muscles of our pelvis, torso and legs constantly stabilize us and ensure we do not fall or move. These muscles do not move much, rather they act in specific muscle contractions. If the contractions do not vary over time, the muscles begin to get tired and weaken. In addition, relative weakness of the muscles or incorrect posture causes the pelvis to move forward. In this situation, the abdomen will protrude slightly forward and the weight of the body begins to shift from the muscles that are supposed to absorb it into the pelvic and spinal ligaments. In this situation, the load on the lumbar vertebral joints increases, resulting in back pain.

What can Ben and many others do to help themselves?

There are several ways to reduce back pain while standing:

- **Sitting** for a few seconds allows spacing of the joints between the vertebrae and can reduce pain intensity. If there is no chair available, you can go down to a **squatting position** for a few seconds and then the pain will decrease in a similar way. See Figure 12 below.

- **Walking** in place or walking around a room will cause the muscles to recontract and move the weight load to them, thus relieving the pain as well.

- **Placing** one leg on a small stool.

- **Tightening and tucking the abdomen in** with a slight backward pelvic rotation will ease their pain. See Figure 13 below.

Increasing your awareness of proper posture on a daily basis and strengthening muscles on a regular basis, e.g., strengthening the abdominal and back muscles, may also prevent and minimize pain while standing.

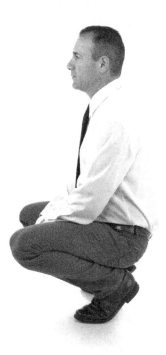

**Figure 12: Squatting position to reduce back pain
while standing**

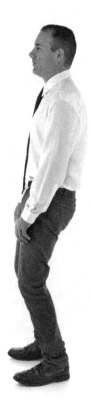

Figure 13: Tightening and tucking the abdomen in to reduce back pain while standing

Learn to Work with your Body Close to Objects

Have you ever seen an arm-wrestling fight? When this is performed amateurishly, there are no clear rules, however the location of the elbow is crucial. The closer the opponent's elbow is to his body, the more power he can generate and the greater his chances of winning the contest. If he cannot move the elbow close to his body, the competitor can bring his whole body closer to his elbow, thereby increasing his chances of winning. Both these examples prove that **performing actions close to the body is more efficient.** This habit should also be applied to our back movements, to save back pain and prevent back problems.

The more actions we take with our hands forward and away from our center of gravity, the greater the burden on our back muscles, ligaments, tendons and discs in the back, thereby increasing the risk of damage. Surgeons, dentists, alternative medicine therapists and hairdressers are an example of professionals who must work diligently to implement this rule. However, working close to our body core is recommended in all daily activities, not just during work hours.

Sometimes I notice my wife or my children squeezing orange juice with a manual juice extractor. "Excellent," I say to myself, "a little extra vitamin C never hurts." However, could they hurt their backs doing this? Hell, yeah! That is because the juicer is not placed near the edge of the kitchen work surface, and close to the body, but rather in the middle of the work surface and far from the body. When I see them do this, I always ask them to bring the juicer closer to them.

In my clinic, there is a wide table with two chairs in front of it with a space in between them. Many times, patients bend over the chair to put their keys and cell phone on the table. They tend to forget that it is better to approach the table from the space between the two chairs, and then place their belongings on the table.

These are examples of seemingly simple actions that are usually carried out in an unfavorable manner and can occur many times during the day, therefore increasing the chance of back damage. The correct action is to change your habits and maintain correct posture. Although the distance between your body and the object may be small, your profit will be great.

Introducing – The 'Sumo Stance'

Have you ever watched a Sumo wrestling contest? In this sport which originated in Japan, two athletes wrestle each other, and one way to win is to push the other participant out of the ring. The wrestler must attempt to maintain stability, so as not to be pushed out of the ring. How does he manage to do this? He must create a wide-base stance.

This stance allows him to be more stable and to use his strong leg muscles to continue the exhausting battle. Although our back is not in an exhausting and difficult situation every day such as in a Sumo contest, even day-to-day activities that are done incorrectly can damage our backs. Therefore, changing our postural habits can help us improve our health.

A 'Sumo Stance' which includes the **spread and bend of legs while standing**, can minimize low back pain and prevent new problems from forming. See Figure 14 below. When should you use this 'Sumo Stance'? For many years, I have been swimming at a local pool. After swimming, I go to the locker room and notice the men who are washing their faces and shaving. They stand in front of the sink with their feet relatively close to each other, with straight legs and locked knees. In addition, they bend over forward with a rounded back to wash their face and shave. These actions are being performed incorrectly, with large loads being transferred to the lower back which can cause damage.

A 'Sumo Stance', with its slight spread and bend of the legs, can help them greatly and can be done when we need to lean the upper body forward. Other times this can be helpful are when we want to pick up a baby out of bed, unload dishes from the dishwasher, or even during a birthday celebration when you lift the child high on his chair. It is recommended to stand with a slightly wide stance and bend the knees slightly.

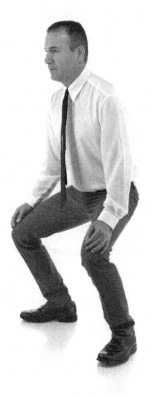

Figure 14: 'Sumo Stance'

Learn to Work with Your Body Facing Objects

You probably have had the opportunity to see at least one Judo fight. Have you noticed the tremendous passion with which the contestants have to bring each other down? In a contest that is so exhausting and physically difficult, the participant knows that he must utilize his physical abilities in the best possible way. One of the ways is to focus on a target and to be in front of it and facing it at all times. Standing facing the opponent allows the participant to use his muscles more effectively to win the fight.

Standing in front of and facing an object allows us to work with our bodies more symmetrically and in a more balanced manner, therefore using our muscles more efficiently thereby reducing the chances of damage to our bodies.

Today, for example, many people order products on the Internet. All these products are sent to us in cardboard boxes, placed next to the door or on the floor of our home. Would you consider standing beside the box and picking it up? This can cause damage to our back. **It is better to stand in front of the box, facing it, approach it and lift it up.**

Standing in front of and facing the box, before lifting it, will allow the leg muscles to act symmetrically and prevent an unequal load on the back muscles. This is easy to perform but entails awareness of how we should work correctly with our body.

A more difficult task, which many of us fail to do correctly, is taking a baby in and out of a car. This task requires bending the body, plus twisting and the lifting of the baby. These actions significantly increase the risk of back injury. Sometimes one mistake is enough to cause injury, and sometimes loads accumulate by repeated incorrect actions, resulting in serious injury.

How do you think you can put a baby into his car seat without damaging your back? The goal, as stated, is to be in front of and facing the object. So my recommendation is to put **one foot in the car in front of and facing the baby's seat while** the second leg remains outside the vehicle, close to the car. **We are applying two methods: One, a wide-standing base, the 'Sumo Stance', and the other, facing the object.** This technique will maintain a healthier back and allow you to enjoy a better quality of life.

I recommend you try to be in front of and facing an object even in the simplest of actions, not necessarily lifting different things - for example, pushing a child on a swing. Many parents stand to the side of the swing, holding the ropes and swinging the child. Again, as far as the back is concerned, this is not symmetrical work; you are not in front of and facing the object and this certainly does not benefit the back. It is best to stand behind the swing, legs slightly spread, which guarantees a perfect and stable activity.

Push or Pull – Which is Best?

Gaby, the Moving Man's Back Problem - A Case Study.

Gaby is a young man in his mid-twenties. Recently he began working in transportation and home moving. Five days a week, Gaby and his fellow workmates transfer the contents of apartments from one place to another.

A week after he started work, Gaby began to complain of pains in the middle of his back and between the shoulder blades which caused him great discomfort during work. Upon examination, the most prominent finding was the restricted movement of the fourth and fifth thoracic vertebrae with stiffness in the mid-back area and lack of flexibility. I explained that a combination of treatments at my clinic and a change in his work habits would be significant in his healing process.

Gaby underwent treatments that included specific vertebrae mobility methods, mobilization and manipulations, accompanied by tailored flexibility and muscle strengthening exercises. During the course of treatment, I explained that the nature of his work which requires lifting and moving objects from place to place for many hours every day, is a danger to his spine and back, and he must therefore adapt new habits. I instructed Gaby to try and reduce the amount of time he walked holding objects in his hands, to use a trolley, and even use a crane to lift the contents directly to the apartment, especially in a building without elevators or in a building where the elevator or stairs are too narrow to carry the furniture.

Gaby underwent a series of treatments at my clinic and changed his work habits. His condition improved beyond recognition. Since then, Gaby advises his co-workers and helps them work more efficiently with their bodies to avoid problems.

●●●

Gaby and his co-workers are not the only ones who need to consider the issue of how to move objects from place to place. Most of us use a cart while shopping to collect items and products before reaching the checkout. Separately, we often need to move a bed or sofa to clean the floor.

Many patients ask me how to perform these tasks correctly. Should we push a cart full of objects, or is it better to, maybe, pull the cart behind us? Which is best? Push or pull? As I mentioned earlier, you must try to work wisely. One way is to use the muscles in your legs to minimize back pain.

Our legs can help us a lot more when we push a cart than if we pull the cart. Our bodies move symmetrically forward, pushing the cart with both our hands - which is actually another advantage. By pulling the loaded cart or pulling a bed out as we step back, our backs are much more bent than in pushing actions, and when combined with the rotation of the head and neck to watch our step as we move backwards, our backs are more vulnerable to damage. When we pull a cart with only one hand behind us while moving forward, the hand, the shoulder blade and the neck on the pulling side are under larger biomechanical loads than when pushing objects, thus exposing them to greater harm.

Another advantage of pushing objects, apart from protecting the back, is that by pushing objects, it is almost impossible to accidentally run over our feet since we are behind the object. There is a higher chance of collision or stubbing our toes using a pulling action.

To summarize, it is preferable to **push** objects, not pull, and of course, use wheels to move objects whenever possible.

Knee Bending as a Method to Prevent and Reduce the Risk of Back Pain

Our backs work very hard during the day. Many spinal movements are performed poorly and expose the spine to damage. Often, damage occurs before the onset of pain, and the wise choice is to prevent back pain and to reduce pain as soon as possible, if any occurs.

One of the most important sources of our strength is the leg muscles, and our proactive and conscious use of them can significantly reduce back loads. The quadriceps, located at the front of the thigh and extending down to the knee, are some of the most powerful muscles in the body, and by activating them, we can prevent back pain.

When you want to get in or out of the car, wash dishes, shave, or pick up any object from the floor, you should **bend your knees and transfer weight to the front of the thigh.** The muscles will absorb the load, resulting in less pressure on discs and other anatomical structures in the back. See Figure 15 below. It is preferable to experience a few temporary muscle pains in the thigh as a result of bending the knees, rather than increase the probability of disc problems, if the knees are locked (i.e., straight).

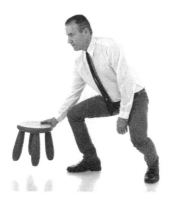

**Figure 15: Knee bending and weight transfer to the front
thigh as a way to prevent back pain**

If you want to lift a light object, such as a pencil, paper, fork, etc.,
you can bend one knee. But if you are lifting a large, heavy and
even wide object, it is recommended to bend both knees. Some
will find it more convenient to bend one or both knees when the
legs are more or less parallel to each other, and some prefer to
place one foot slightly forward. .

I can tell you with certainty that people who suffer acute back
pain and sometimes even chronic pain may experience a stronger
back pain if they do not bend one or both knees to perform one
of the tasks described above.

Another advantage to bending the knees is that the pelvis usually
rotates backwards, (similar to bringing the knees toward the
chest, while laying down on your back,) causing the vertebrae
to move slightly apart from each other, thus relieving back pain.

In my personal experience, after many years of adhering to
this concept, applying this principle is **vitally important** in
maintaining back health.

Learn to Minimize Forward Inclination of the Torso or Bending Your Torso While Standing

I am sure that you have seen images or heard about the famous Leaning Tower of Pisa. This tower, located in the city of Pisa, Italy, is famous for sideways inclination thereby attracting many people to see it, from all over the world. A fact that most people do not know is that for years the tower has continued to tilt further and further. The angle of the tilt increases a little each year, until its collapse is inevitable!

As an expert on spinal problems, I often use this example in my lectures because it perfectly simulates the importance of erect posture. The spine often acts in the same way as the Tower of Pisa, and the more time we spend in leaning the torso forwards or bending it, the more likely we are to suffer damage.

Most of us tilt our backs forward for too long in performing basic activities such as cleaning the table, shaving, brushing teeth, changing bedding and making the bed, removing a garment from a low shelf in the closet, bathing children in the bathtub and many other activities that are performed in non-optimal posture that can result in spinal damage. These repetitive acts of tilting and bending forward increase pressure and weight loads on back muscles, ligaments of the spine and pelvis, and on the intervertebral discs, even if no pain is initially experienced. See Figure 16 below.

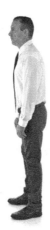

Figure 16: The forward tilt of the torso increases the load on the back

As the forward tilt of the back increases, the chances of damage to anatomical structures becomes greater, and the muscles will have to work harder to prevent our fall.

Many people suffer from various disc and spinal narrowing canal problems. For many, the body tends to tilt or bend forward, making daily functioning difficult, which is then accompanied by great suffering. Therefore, when you want to do actions in front of your body, you should be aware of maintaining correct posture, minimizing the tilt of the torso as far as possible, getting as close to the object as possible, bending one or both knees, standing with your legs apart and, if necessary, inclining your back forward, rather than bending and arching it.

In addition, regular and corrective action to strengthen the back muscles, along with initiating a backward motion of the vertebral joints (and not bending), will also help maintain proper posture and reduce the possibility of developing a non-erect posture similar to the Tower of Pisa.

Learn How to Prevent or Reduce Back Pain in the Gym

As a child, I loved sports, so it only seemed natural that as soon as I finished my compulsory national service, I attended the Wingate Institute for physical education where I studied posture training and preventive exercises. It was here that I acquired the fundamentals of correct posture and correct general body movement. During this time, I also became a certified a gym instructor. Why am I telling you this? Because today many teenagers and adults are aware of the importance of keeping their bodies in healthy condition, and many choose to workout at the gym. Improper training in the gym can lead to major back pain. Therefore, focusing on correct posture during exercising and workouts is vitally important.

Here are some tips to help you look after your back while at the gym:

- **Standing and not sitting.** It is advisable, as much as possible, to perform muscle strengthening exercises such as lifting weights **in a standing position.** The pressure on the intervertebral disc is greater when sitting, which increases the likelihood of back pain.

- Minimizing **the tilting forward of the back** while sitting and standing, and to **keep the back straight** while lifting weights.

- **Reducing distance.** It is best to lift a weight **as close to the body as possible**. An example of the application of these principles is, in order to strengthen the biceps in the front arm, stand with your back straight and supported against the wall, knees slightly bent, legs apart, and a weight in the palm of your hand - a straight arm, **elbow close to the body**. The exercise is to bend the elbow and straighten the hand back. Perform this exercise several times and change hands.

- **Balanced muscle strengthening**. One of the most common back-pain-causing problems seen at a gym, is muscle imbalance between the muscles at the front of the body and the muscles at the back of the body. Many gym-goers like to strengthen the abdominal and chest muscles at the front of the body, neglecting or only slightly strengthening back muscles.

Remember, the back has many muscles, some of which function differently than to the chest and abdominal muscles. Prolonged activation of the front muscles, along with inadequate operation of the back muscles (as seen in most cases), can cause problems in the lower back, shoulder blades and neck. It is advised to ensure that gym activity combines exercises for both the front and back of our bodies, thus avoiding injuries and the development of muscle imbalance.

Applying these principles is significant in maintaining our backs in general, not just in the gym. It is always advisable to consult with a professional prior to commencing the activity.

118 | Dr. Ronen Welgrin

Lifting and Putting Down Objects

The Correct Order of Movement to Prevent Back Damage

One of the major dangers to the spine, neck and back is lifting objects incorrectly. Sometimes a small error in lifting an object can cause significant back damage. In most cases, pain will not be experienced by lifting the wrong way occasionally, but the damage nevertheless is being done.

If you continue to lift in the wrong way, pain will arise and serious damage can be caused to muscles, ligaments and discs. Therefore, it is vitally important to know and apply the principles of lifting and placing objects correctly.

1. **The weight of the object**. First, understand which kind of object you wish to lift. If it is too heavy, call for help.

2. **Check the area**. Check that the area where the object is located is free from any obstructions that can interfere with you lifting it. Also, check the area in which you want to place the object for similar obstacles.

3. **Stand facing the object.** Approach the object you want to lift and stand in front of it, facing it.

4. **'Sumo Stance'.** Bend your knees and slightly spread your legs. Try not to bend your neck and back.

5. **Symmetrical hold.** Hold the object with both hands.

6. **Lift the object and hold it close to your body.** Lift it up and bring it closer to you.

7. **Straighten your back.** Stand up, straighten your legs and push against the floor with your feet.

8. **Minimize the time you hold an object and lower it safely.** At this stage, when the object is being held in your hands and you are standing, try to minimize the time you hold the object and find the nearest location to place the object. Never lower the object while rotating your body.

9. **Follow the same procedure when you want to place the object.** Move closer and stand in front of the location where you wish to place the object, with your legs slightly apart. Bend your knees without twisting and bending your neck and back. Put the object down. Straighten up again by straightening your legs and pushing against the floor with your feet.

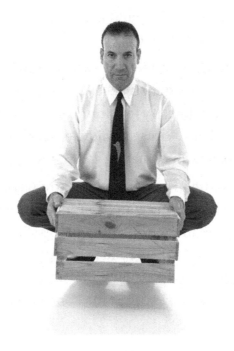

Figure 17: Picking up and placing objects correctly

Sometimes You Have to Ask for Help –A Case Study

It was Wednesday, my day off, the day I tried to spend more time with my immediate family. I picked up my two children from their acrobatics class and took them home. My wife asked me to pick up some shopping. It was 7:30 in the evening so I decided to stop off at a local shop, made my selection and went to wait in line at the checkout.

As I waited in line, I heard the cashier, a young woman, asking the customer in front of her to put the apples he had bought on the scale. Although she should have done this herself, her request seemed logical to me, since his bag was full. Then, to my great surprise, the young cashier asked him to put all his other purchases on the scale, one after the other.

When the man had finished putting every bag in turn on the scale, he asked the cashier why she had not done it herself. The cashier looked into his eyes and replied with a smile that she did not want to injure her back!

The rest of the people in the line continued in the same manner. When it came to my turn, besides helping her, I congratulated her for her courage and her awareness of back problem prevention.

●●●

If you do repetitive actions that could expose your back to damage or injury, there is no shame asking for help from others!

My Grandparents' Pulley

I remember that when I was a little boy, every Saturday we would visit my grandparents, Grandpa Yermiyahu and Grandma Rivka Welgrin, who lived on the fourth floor of an apartment building.

For elderly people, going up and down stairs several times a day is not a simple task especially if they like to go out or if they have shopping to take home from the supermarket. Their backs, arms and legs are prone to tire quickly, and aches and pains begin to appear. The solution my grandparents found was very creative! They put a cable in place that extends from the fourth floor to the entrance of the building with a pulley attached. At the end of the cable, they attached a hook, to which they tied a strong basket where they placed their shopping bags. When they reached their apartment, they then pulled the shopping bags up using the cable, saving them from carrying the bags that otherwise could have affected their backs and increased the likelihood of damage.

Even today, many people still do not make enough use of **wheels** to move objects from place to place. Shopping carts are a significant tool, but some people still prefer to carry groceries with their hands, and that is a shame. It is better to walk with a cart **through** the supermarket, and after having paid at the checkout, to walk with your purchases **in** the cart to your car.

Proper postural awareness and intelligent body behavior can prevent a lot of bodily damage.

Which Object Should be Picked Up First?

After a day at the clinic, I go to the car and put my personal things inside: my cell phone, my wallet and a bag that contains my laptop. After a short drive, I park the car next to my house and then get out of the car to pick up my belongings.

This is the stage where most people make a mistake! People do not know which object they should pick up first, and which object should be the last. The ideal scenario is to try to **bend as little as possible** while holding a heavy object, in order to prevent back problems. Do not forget that after a long day at work, your body is tired, and therefore more vulnerable and prone to damage. It is well worth investing more thought in your movements, to reduce the probability of damage.

In the scenario I described above, **you should remove the bag containing the laptop, which is the heaviest object, last.** The first objects to be picked up should be the cellphone and wallet. They should be taken out and placed in your pocket while standing and only then should you bend down to carefully and correctly remove the bag with the laptop. Selecting the order of removing items from the car can save your back and neck from problems later on.

There are situations in life where we are required to pick up a heavy object and walk with it a certain distance until we reach our destination. It could be a small but heavy bag or a full shopping bag or any other object.

Let's say, for example, you want to get into a vehicle while carrying something. Most people prefer to get into a car by bending their body with the object in their hands. This causes substantial weight loads on the muscles, ligaments and discs in the lower back, and can cause them considerable damage.

To ease pressure on the back and its various parts, I recommend that you **first place the object in the vehicle while standing,** and only afterwards, once your hands are free, you can seat yourself safely without causing any damage to your back.

How to Reduce or Prevent Back Pain While Placing Your Infant in a Car?

Parents with small children must place and remove their kids from their car seat on a daily basis, and often several times a day. Grandparents who try to help out with their grandchildren are also faced with this issue. The question is how to do this correctly so as not to damage the back and spine. Their main mistake is that they first bend their head and body into the vehicle while their feet stay out of the car, on the road or pavement. Such actions, often done incorrectly, increase the chances of back pain and actual damage later on. Changing habits and being aware of proper posture can significantly reduce the chance of damage. So how do you place a baby into the car seat without causing damage to your back?

First, it is best to position the stroller as close to the vehicle door as possible. Then, while the baby is still in the stroller and you have locked the wheels to prevent slipping, open the back door of the vehicle and make sure that the seat is free from objects, properly positioned and secured. At the same time, ensure that the floor of the vehicle is free from any objects. Only then should you lift the baby from the stroller and hold him close to your body. If the baby seat is on the right-hand side, get as close to it as you can and put your right foot inside the vehicle, facing the baby seat. Bend your right knee, put your body and your head in, keeping your back as straight as possible, with the baby still in your hands and close to your body.

Tilt your torso a little forward so your body weight is placed mostly on the right thigh muscle, above the bent knee. See Figure 18 below. Place the baby safely in the seat, strap him in, and then remove your body from the vehicle, bringing your foot out last.

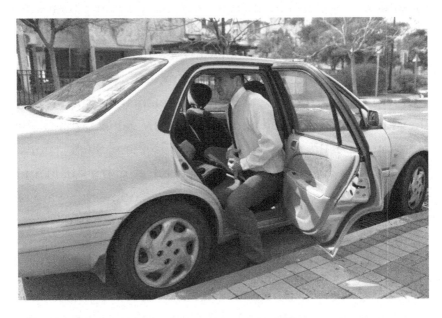

Figure18: Placing and securing your infant in the car seat in the right position

Symmetry: Use Both Sides of the Body

Preventing Back Problems with Symmetrical Effort

The human body is relatively symmetrical. We have two hands, two legs, a symmetrical face, and so on. However, the symmetry is not absolute. The heart is located behind and slightly to the left of the breastbone, the liver is located on the right side of the abdomen, and our function, too, is not symmetrical. For example, we use our more dominant hand (left or right) to lift, drag, push, and pull different objects. Some of us are in continuous non-symmetrical positions in which we bend to one side or repeated actions of bending and twisting of the spine to one side, much more than the other side, especially during work. Production line workers in factories, and dentists are good examples.

Consider a tennis player. Do you think that a tennis player will strengthen only the same side of the body as the hand he holds the racquet with when he goes to the gym? Of course not! The more our body is in an asymmetrical state, the greater the chances of exposure to damage.

Cases such as a short leg, e.g., an anatomical condition since birth in which the legs are not the same length, or one flat foot (congenital or acquired) compared to the other foot, can cause an unbalanced pelvis. In these cases, walking will not be symmetrical and there may be a slight limp. The spine is then more exposed to muscle, ligament, and disc injuries. An insole, and sometimes an orthotic aid, may provide a solution to these problems.

Many people leave the shopping center with full bags in only one hand, usually their dominant hand. They walk like this to their car and load the bags all at once, with a slight swing to put them on the backseat or inside the trunk. This entire process involving bending and turning the back to one side, combined with excessive weight on the same side, is not good for one's back, and can even cause pain and damage.

It is much better to carry the bags with both hands, dividing the load as equally as possible, and instead of swinging them all at once into the vehicle, place the bags one by one.

Another example: most children carry their school bag on one shoulder, and usually on the same shoulder, for many years. This results in increased stress on muscles and nerves in that area and can cause pain. These asymmetrical operations continue for many years. Later on as adults, these children tend to carry heavy bags (such as on a family trip), on the same side that they used to carry their backpacks on, the same side that been exposed to damage for many years.

Therefore, it is really no wonder that many adults complain of neck pain, pain in their shoulders and shoulder blades, and even pain in their hands, numbness, etc. Carrying a backpack on both shoulders allows better load distribution on anatomical structures in the back and reduces the risk of future damage.

To summarize, symmetrical function will allow our bodies to function better, prevent and even save us from back pain. There is, therefore, a need for structural and functional symmetry to prevent future spine and back problems.

Recommended Places to Sit in a Banquet Hall

You enter a banquet hall, there is no set seating arrangement and you can choose where you would like to sit. What seat should you choose? Is there a seat that can reduce and even prevent back and neck pain more than other seats or placements? Most people do not have a special preference as to where they sit, but most prefer to sit next to friends or family, which is fine of course.

Personally, I believe that choosing a place to sit is significant, and I always try to find seating where the chance of damaging my back is minimal. The truth is that it is very easy, since I may be the only person who thinks about the aspect of finding a place to sit where I can enjoy the event, while at the same time prevent back and neck pain.

In order to know where these places are, we must find out where the main celebration area is and try to be in front of it, rather than to the side of it. The dance floor is the main focal point and the eyes of the guests are directed there most of the time. Therefore, when I choose a place to sit, I will always choose a chair located directly in front of and facing the dance floor. It does not have to be near the dance floor, as long as it is facing it. This choice of seating ensures my spine, back, neck and head are straight in front of the dance floor, **without** the need of having to **twist and turn**.

Many people sit with their backs to the dance floor or to the side of it, then bend and twist their neck and back to one side to see what is happening there. They may sit there for a few hours, with intervals between their asymmetrical postures. Is it any wonder then that later that day, or the next day, they encounter neck or back pain?

If you arrive late and there are only a few seats vacant that do not meet the criteria I mentioned earlier, I always recommended rotating your chair, so that it faces the dance floor.

It is worth remembering that small, accumulated trauma to the back, even without current pain, can eventually cause great damage accompanied by great suffering. Therefore, it is important to maintain proper posture and symmetrical functioning with our bodies as much as possible.

The Common Mistake
of Amateur Swimmers, Swimming
the Front Crawl Stroke

When I was 10 years old, we were sent as a class to swimming lessons at the local swimming pool. I remember the instructor asking each of us to swim about ten meters so that he could put us in the right group according to our swimming ability. I tried to swim the front crawl stroke, a fairly uncoordinated effort, including slapping the water with my hands. I was sent to Group C for children who really had no idea how to swim, while most of my friends were put in the A Group.

The feeling of frustration and disappointment accompanied me for many years. At the age of twenty-two, when I was a physical education student, I decided to register for a lifeguard course. Throughout the course, I did not meet even the minimum time required to pass the exams. The training was difficult. My classmates passed the test with ease. My father, as I recall, was the only parent who came to cheer his son on the day of the exam. His loud voice of encouragement helped me, reach the minimum required for the first time and I passed the exam.

Make no mistake, I am not a great swimmer. But to be a lifeguard, and even to earn a bit of extra cash many years ago, I did succeed at swimming. Since then I have been swimming a mile twice a week, and this is another of the many precautions I take to prevent back pain.

So what is the common mistake of amateur swimmers swimming the front crawl stroke? Turning the head and breathing to the same side all the time, an action that creates asymmetrical movements in the neck, combined with uneven loads on anatomical structures on both sides of the neck and back. It is recommended to breathe once to the right and once to the left.

Sitting

The Negative Effects Prolonged Sitting Has on the Body

Today, more than ever, we are witnessing a growing phenomenon: the amount of time we sit in a day. Our dependence on computers, found in almost every home and workplace, require us to use them more frequently and for a longer duration. Our dependence on computers in many workplaces is growing, and more and more workers are required to operate them - while sitting of course. Additionally, we spend more time watching television and suffer longer commuting times than ever before.

People become less mobile and spend more time sitting, which can lead to serious health consequences. Sitting for many hours during the day, for years, can cause slower body metabolism, obesity, decreased functioning of the cardiac system, increased blood pressure, and disturbances in blood supply to the legs and back to the heart. As a result, various diseases may arise, which could have been avoided if we were more physically active.

During prolonged sitting, the burden on the pelvic bones increases and the leg bones are relatively inactive. Therefore, in prolonged sitting conditions, leg bones become weak, their density decreases, and the likelihood of future damage increases. Leg muscles do not function properly due to prolonged sitting, and will not be able to function optimally later when we need to perform various tasks such as carrying objects, lifting a baby out of the car, or running several kilometers.

In order to minimize back pain and prevent new back problems, leg muscles should be used often. Even if they are slightly weakened due to insufficient exercise as a result of prolonged or cumulative sitting, the chances of spine and back damage increase.

Therefore, it is advisable to engage in more physical activity. If you are prone to long periods of sitting, get up occasionally and activate your body. We did not evolve to be 'couch potatoes'.

The Negative Effects Prolonged Sitting has on the Back

Prolonged sitting with few breaks, whether at home or at work, is not recommended for our spine. Sitting for long periods may cause lack of movement in the vertebrae thereby accelerating the degenerative changes that can occur in them. These changes can be described as 'rusting of the joints' of the vertebrae and can include the appearance of bone spurs, i.e., bony protrusions that emerge from the vertebrae. Vertebral movement will gradually decrease due to these degenerative changes, and back pain will begin to appear.

The vertebrae, in most cases, bend over while sitting, similar to a spring, bent and arched forward, thus being compressed at their front portion. This speeds up the appearance of degenerative processes in the vertebrae.

Sitting, especially in a bent or slumped position, causes the ligaments of the vertebrae to lengthen, stretch and weaken. The ligaments gradually lose their ability to provide stability to the vertebrae and to the vertebral joints and can be a possible additional source of pain.

In a similar way, the back muscles also lengthen and weaken. Their lack of motion and sitting in a slumped position rather than in optimal sitting postures increase the chances of muscle pain and muscle stiffness.

Prolonged sitting also does not benefit the **intervertebral discs.** The discs begin to compress, become thinner and lose their main ability to function in absorbing the shocks and loads that are applied to the vertebrae. The compression of the discs due to the weight of the upper body, along with slouched sitting, causes compression in the front part of the discs, thus causing them to protrude or herniate at the rear part. See Figure 19 below. A protruding disc or disc herniation can cause local back pain, or even radiation to the limbs, hands or feet, and cause symptoms such as numbness, 'shooting pains', muscle aches and muscle weakness.

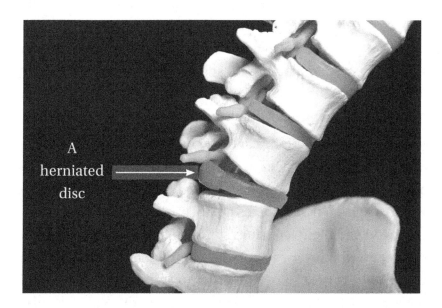

Figure 19: A plastic model that demonstrates a bending forward of the vertebrae and backward herniation of the disc

Learn to Reduce Your Sitting Time

As previously mentioned, sitting has many negative effects, and one of the main goals in reducing back pain and prevent new spinal problems is to reduce the amount of time you sit. People whose work involves prolonged sitting need to get up often from the chair, if they can, take a walk to the next room, a stroll down the hallway, and even perform some flexibility and strengthening exercises, if time and place permitting. If you do not have enough time and you cannot take a few minutes' walk, you can even stand still, walk in place, or do some standing exercises. Today there are also stand-up computer desks, an additional aid that can assist in easing back damage.

If you are planning a long car trip, you should stop on the way at organized parking places or gas stations and leave your car for a few minutes to rest your neck, stretch your legs, and of course your back, even if these areas do not hurt! If you have planned a train ride or a flight, consider sitting on the aisle. This way you can get up whenever you feel like, without having to disturb the people sitting next to you, in order to stand up or take a stroll down the aisle. If you are on a plane, walk to the end of the aisle where there is usually more room for you to perform several exercises for your legs, back, neck and shoulders.

The Hotel's Stand-Up Computer Station - A Case Study

One of the most enjoyable family trips I remember was to the Black Forest in Germany, during the children's school holiday. We had an amazing time there. On the last day of our vacation, we decided to drive across the border and stay in a hotel near the airport in France since we had an early morning flight back home.

Not far from the reception desk, my son spotted a mounted computer screen showing various fun and challenging games for children and youth, so you can imagine that it immediately intrigued him and he went to check it out.

He played the various games standing up, not sitting down, and as I watched him, I thought to myself what a great idea it was and how easily it could be applied in many other places so that children would spend less time sitting down, thus improving their back health.

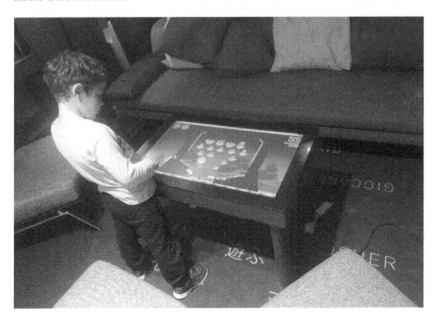

Figure 20: Stand-Up Computer Station

Try to Sit Straight and Not Slouch

Slouched sitting does not require any body effort. Bent and convex sitting eliminates the lumbar arch. Most people adopt this way of sitting because it is easier, does not involve using the muscles and because they are unaware of correct posture. Slouched sitting causes more pressure on the vertebrae and discs, and increases the probability of damage. Even if you sit with a slouched back and do not feel any pain, the damage may already be occurring.

An easy test may be performed to confirm if you sit in a slouched or upright position. If while sitting, you are able to insert the palm of your hand between the back of the chair and your lower back, then you are sitting upright. If you find that you are unable to do this, it means you are sitting in a slouched position.

Although this is not easy, try to sit upright. Sometimes, back muscles are too weak to hold our torso in an upright position. In this case, we will find ourselves slouching and sitting with a bent back. Sometimes, because of an activity the body is not accustomed to, sitting upright may cause slight muscle pain. The main thing is not to give up - new habits are hard to adopt. Sometimes it takes time for the body and the back to adapt to new habits. Most importantly, sitting upright, as explained above, reduces the likelihood of future back injury. See Figure 21 below.

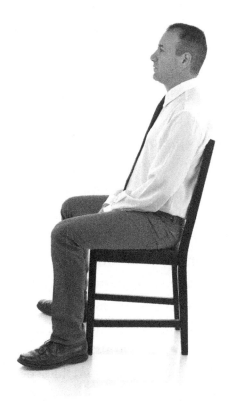

Figure 21: Sitting upright

The Effect Electric Bicycles have on Backs

This new craze that started a few years ago has rapidly gained popularity. During the last few years, millions of people have chosen to use electric bicycles for their transportation needs, with these figures rising each year. Many teenagers and adults now hardly walk at all, let alone walk the recommended daily distance, and prefer to ride electric bikes to reach their destinations. Most electric bicycle users prefer to use the accelerator lever, instead of pedaling with their legs, meaning even less exercise!

People ride these bikes for quite some time each day, usually with a bent back, which may result in various possibilities of back damage, especially for teenage cyclists who start from an early age. Pedaling helps to absorb shocks that may be caused from the riding surface and penetrate from the body of the bicycle down to the cyclist's legs and up the spine. However, in most cases, the cyclist sits in a static position, without using his legs, meaning that the lower limb muscles cannot absorb the shocks to them. The result is overload and shocks reaching the spine and back that may result in damage. You should consider minimizing cycling time on electric bikes, and when riding, try pedaling and refrain from sitting in a bent position.

Use Lower Back Support to Reduce and Prevent Pain

Maintaining the natural lumbar curve is a significant goal, and requires great effort. This is not an easy task, especially for people who tend to sit for many hours a day.

Sometimes we lack the strength required to work the muscles and maintain an erect posture in our lower back while sitting, and need aids that will make the task of keeping our back in an optimal position possible. For example, on trains, buses, and in airplanes, the seats cannot be adjusted in an ideal way, so it is more difficult to maintain the natural curve of the lower back vertebrae. However, you can use a support such as a small cushion, rolled piece of clothing or small towel that you can place behind your lower back to keep your natural lumbar curve. See Figure 22 below. Sometimes, an adjustable chair may be used which also lends support to the lower back.

Lower back support allows the vertebrae and discs to be in a position that is almost the same as their normal state, thus minimizing the chance of future damage.

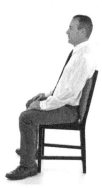

Figure 22: Use a lower back support

Learn to Use Your Hands While Sitting to Avoid Back Pain

If you suffer from low back pain and must sit for prolonged periods of time, it is a good idea to use your hands to help you absorb part of the pressure .The goal is to try and reduce as much pressure from the vertebrae and discs and using your hands will help to ease the load.

First, place your forearms on the table in front of you while sitting, move your body weight slightly forward and lean on your forearms. Leaning on your forearms or elbows allows you to keep a straight back more easily, thus saving back pain. See Figure 23 below. If you suffer from severe back pain and find you have considerable difficulty sitting down in or getting up from the chair, you can place both palms on the chair, one on each side of the body to push yourself up, which also reduces pressure on the vertebrae and the intervertebral discs. See Figure 24 below.

You can use these two methods even if you do not have any back pain, and just want to reduce the probability of suffering from pain in the future. Sometimes, due to general tiredness, especially in the back, we tend to sit in a slouched position or tend to lounge in a chair. This is when back damage can increase. Therefore, the use of our hands, as described above, can effectively assist in preventing back damage.

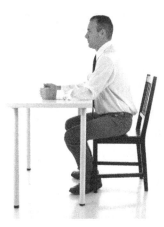

Figure 23: Leaning on the forearms and elbows as a way to reduce and prevent back problems

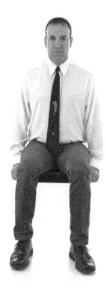

Figure 24: Placing palms on the chair and leaning on them as a way to reduce and prevent back problems

Learn How to Reduce Back Pain While Sitting on a Sofa

Sometimes after a day at work, our body is tired, and all we want to do is take a rest. A favorite option for many people is the sofa in the living room, because they can choose to sit or lie down. Lying on your **side** on the sofa can reduce pressure on the vertebrae due to the horizontal position of the spine, rather than a vertical one.

If you like to sit on the sofa, to watch TV or talk with friends, the way you sit requires different evaluations. The main problem is that most sofas are **too soft, causing the buttocks and pelvis to sag and slightly rotate backwards** (see the importance of the pelvis as described in the beginning of the book in basic concepts), therefore creating greater pressure on the ligaments, muscles and discs, **and increase the probability of damage**. See Figure 25 below.

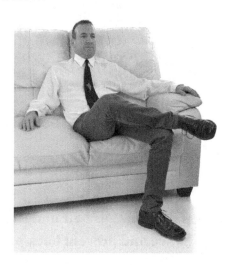

Figure 25: Incorrect sitting position on a sofa or soft surface

The softer the surface we sit on, the more difficult it will be to maintain the natural lumbar curve, which may lead to an increase in the probability of back damage. Knowing how to sit properly on a soft platform is something everyone should know in order to avoid and prevent spinal damage. Most people tend to sit **on the middle of the sofa** in a slouched position, while leaning back on the sofa to support the shoulder blades. In this position, the pelvis rotates backwards, the lumbar vertebrae are straightened and the risk of back damage increases. Some of us also partially straighten our legs. In this situation, the hamstring muscles in the back of the thighs begin to stretch, leading to a worsening backward pelvic rotation, sinking back on the couch, and an increase in the likelihood of pain and/or injury.

The solution **is not to straighten your legs, but to try to sit upright**, which requires awareness. See Figure 26 below. The problem is that sitting in this position for a length of time is difficult. Another option is to place a cushion behind the middle of your back and against the sofa back; this will prevent the pelvis from rotating backwards and allow the back muscles a little rest.

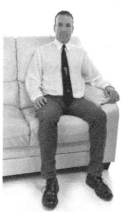

Figure 26: Correct Sitting. Option A: Sitting upright on the middle of the sofa cushion, knees bent

Another seating option is to **sit back on the sofa and place a cushion for support** on the lower back. This position is good for the back, but can cause the legs to straighten partially, creating pressure and discomfort on the gastrocnemius muscles under the knees, in the upper calves, against the sofa. See Figure 27 below.

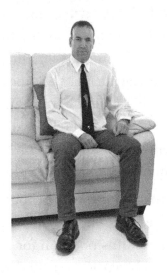

Figure 27: Correct Sitting. Option B: Sitting on the back of the sofa, while using a pillow

Another possibility is to **sit on the front edge of the sofa, where the seat is firmer, again, with a straight back.** Moving the feet back in this sitting position can help us stay in this position longer, with minimal damage to the back. See Figure 28 below.

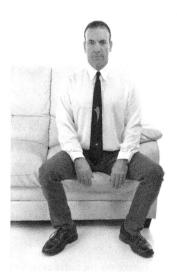

Figure 28: Correct Sitting. Option C: Sitting on the front edge of the sofa

To summarize, you can choose to sit in the front, middle or back of the sofa. If you find this uncomfortable, it is possible, and even better, to sit on a regular chair.

In Which Pocket Should you Keep your Wallet?

Have you ever driven a car when one of its tires has less air than the others? The feeling is uncomfortable and it feels like the car's grip on the road is not good. Over time, tires wear and the weight of the car is not evenly distributed, causing the engine to work harder and a rise in fuel consumption. In short, the vehicle is not balanced!

This is exactly what happens to us when we sit on a wallet in the back pocket of our pants. The pelvis is unbalanced, one side is compressed more than the other, the wallet causes pressure on muscles and nerves and can cause local pain in the buttocks or lower back, or even radiate pain to the back or outer leg, sometimes causing a feeling of numbness in the legs.

In most cases, people (mostly men), will not feel pain while sitting on their wallet in a coffee shop or working in the office, especially the first few times. They may feel a little uncomfortable, but not enough to take their wallet out of their pocket.

Most people tend to live by the motto, "If nothing hurts, that means I am healthy", and do not understand that by sitting on their wallet, they are causing damage. For most men, sitting on their wallet is a habit of years, so the chances of damage to their backs increase. This lack of awareness prevents them from maintaining their health.

Therefore, placing items in back pockets while sitting is not recommended, not even a wadded up tissue or handkerchief! Placing such items in **front pockets** can save back problems and can also keep your wallet safe from pickpockets!

Learn to Minimize Lifting Objects While Sitting

Lifting objects is a common daily activity. Many times throughout the day, we are required to pick up things like various bags or different objects while we are seated. Children in school need to pick up their bags which are crammed with books from the floor next to them,. During family meals, we sometimes want to pick up a pot or dish from the table to serve food. Cashiers in shops and factory workers have to repeatedly pick up objects, many times in a sitting position.

Lifting objects while sitting creates a considerable weight load on anatomical structures in the back such as discs, muscles, ligaments and tendons, and can cause them substantial damage. **To reduce the risk of back damage, it is recommended that you avoid lifting objects while sitting.** Instead, get up from your chair and stand up to pick up objects correctly. See Figure 29 below.

Picking up objects when standing allows the leg muscles to contract and help in absorbing the weight load, which is difficult to do while seated.

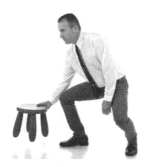

Figure 29: Lifting objects correctly when standing

Implementation of this principle from an early age can reduce the risk of back pain. It is, of course, recommended to be applied at any age. For most people, changing their daily behavioral habits is difficult and they need a wake-up call and a lot of practice in order for these actions to become 'automatic'.

One of the most common mistakes occurs almost every morning when parents take their children to school. In most cases, children get into the car with their bag on their backs and then, after they sit down, they take the bag off their back by bending and twisting their backs.

When they arrive at school, they lift the heavy bag back onto their shoulders while sitting, again bending and twisting the spine. These actions cause unnecessary loads on the back and may increase the chances of pain and future damage. At the end of the school day, some of the parents arrive with their vehicles to pick up their children, and then the same mistakes occur again. It is the responsibility of the adult to explain to children how to best use their bodies in every-day activities. It is advised, for example, to place the bag in the trunk of the car.

How to Get Up from a Chair Without Damaging your Back?

Many people report low back pain especially when they want to change position from sitting to standing. This is not simple when back and spine problems are present, especially among people who suffer from various intervertebral disc problems, such as a protruding or a herniated disc. Proper posture awareness and correct functioning of the legs, back, hands and head can save a great deal of suffering and pain when shifting from a sitting to a standing position. The following points demonstrate how to get up correctly:

1. **Slide Forward.** First, you should slide slowly forward to the edge of the chair. You can use your palms to push against the seat slightly, and keep your back relatively straight.

2. **Spread Your Legs.** In doing so, shift your body weight forward, and with a straight back press against the floor with your feet. If the pain in your back is strong, this movement can be repeated several times so that the leg muscles will be more effective when actually getting up.

3. **Move Body Weight Forward.** While getting up, it is advisable to move your weight forward, towards the front part of your feet. You can gently press your hands on the front thighs.

4. **Getting Up Off A Chair.** While leaning with a straight back forward, bending your knees and buttocks slightly protruding backward, get up from the chair. As you get up from the chair, do not lower your head, and be careful not to arch your spine. See Figures 30 A - D - The stages of correct sitting to standing.

Implementing these steps can save you from unnecessary back pain.

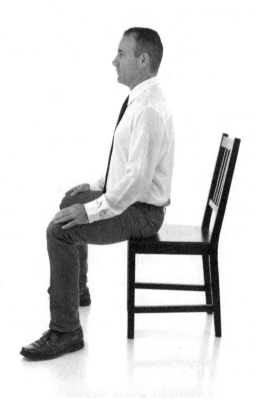

Figure 30 A -B: Sliding forward and legs apart

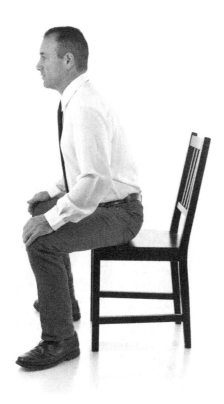

Figure 30 C: Moving the weight forward

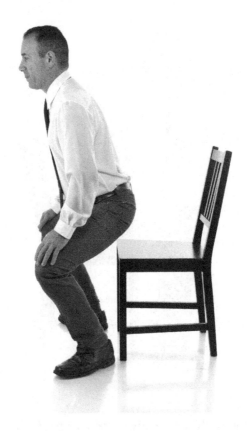

Figure 30 D: Getting up from the chair

Correct Bathroom Posture is Important

Many people suffer from chronic low back pain which becomes especially acute while sitting. Often, the disc in the lower back causes increased pain while sitting, and even the thought of sitting frightens them. This thought occurs, for example, when one has to use the toilet. The problem is that many people think that the toilet is a "place of recreation" where one can sit for a long time with a book or newspaper without anyone interfering them - however this is not the case!

Prolonged sitting, especially in a bent and slouched position while reading, can further aggravate lower back pain for those who already suffer from pain. Therefore, it is advisable to go to the toilet, when you are in real need, minimize the time you sit, and try to sit in an upright position.

Those who suffer from lower back pain can also perform several backward bends with their back before sitting on the toilet. It is also advisable to ensure that the roll of toilet paper is not on the floor but on a holder or in a higher position, for ease of use.

Some people apply too much pressure while going to the toilet, which can further worsen their back pain. You may want to consider gentle and intermittent pressures thus saving a great deal of suffering.

You should maintain a straight back while cleaning yourself, and when you want to stand up, slide your buttocks forward to the front edge of the toilet seat, and get up by pushing against the floor with your feet while keeping your back relatively straight.

It is very possible that you will feel back pain while getting up off the toilet; therefore, it is advisable to be careful and perform gentle backward bends after getting up.

How to Behave with a Disc Problem?

Learn About One of the Main Reasons of Various Disc Problems

One of the most common problems that can cause a great deal of suffering and discomfort relates to poor functioning of the intervertebral disc. The disc is a kind of "pad" between two vertebrae, and its function is to prevent the vertebrae from touching each other. The disc is a fairly round-shaped cartilage tissue, and because of its unique composition, it can change shape and be compresed, due to the load applied to it. When the loads are relieved, the disc can return to its previous shape.

The disc plays a significant role in shock absorbing; without discs, the entire weight load would affect the vertebrae themselves and cause them damage. The disc consists of two parts. The interior, called the nucleus, is gel-like and mostly composed of water, and the outer layer is called the annulus fibrosus. The annulus is thicker, and it surrounds and protects the nucleus. Many disc problems are related to damage to these two parts.

Common causes of disc damage are due to improper posture, back injuries that can happen from car accidents, falls, sharp and abrupt back movements, improperly lifting objects, etc.

Imagine a rubber watering hose lying on the grass. Now try to imagine that you are standing with one foot pressing on the hose. As you do, the diameter of the hose reduces in size, disturbing the optimal flow of water. The same thing happens with a protruding disc or herniated disc which can press on the covers around the spinal cord, and in doing so interferes with the passage of nerve commands throughout the body.

The disc is located on the vertebral body in front of the spinal canal, and in some disc damage, especially a protruding or herniated disc, the result is pressure on the spinal canal and a negative effect on the spinal cord and on the nerves located inside the spinal canal.

One of the most common causes of disc problems is poor posture, especially postures associated with prolonged bending of the lumbar spine, as in slouched sitting. In this situation, the vertebrae are compressed and get closer to each other in their front part, and they open and move away from each other in their rear part. This new opening created at the rear part may allow the disc to protrude where it might touch the nerve and cause severe pain. See Figure 31 below. **Repeated bending of the vertebrae increases the probability of disc damage**, which can be seen as reduced thickness of the disc, thus decreasing its ability to absorb shocks and excess weight, and even a change in the shape of the disc.

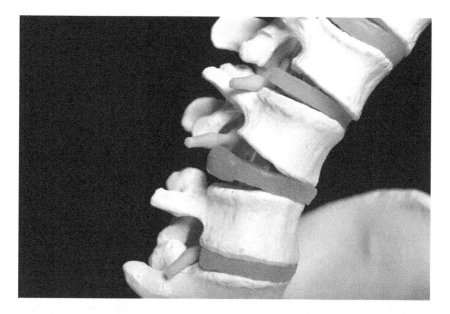

Figure 31: A plastic model of the vertebrae demonstrating a backward protruding disc as a result of a forward bend of the vertebrae

Between each two vertebrae, on the right and on the left, there is an opening called the foraminal canal through which the spinal nerve emerges. Often the canal becomes narrower and this may cause pressure or irritation of the nerve located inside it which then causes severe pain. There are three main reasons for this. The first is that disc degeneration causes the vertebrae to get closer to each other, and the diameter of this opening is reduced in its vertical size. The second is the protrusion of a disc, or a herniated disc, backwards and sideways, which can also narrow the canal in the front part and cause nerve pressure. The third reason being that due to poor posture, the intervertebral joints begin to degenerate.

This degeneration is characterized by thickening of the joints and causes the canal to narrow in the rear part. The combination of these factors is frequently seen in X-rays, and shows the narrowing of the canal from several directions causing pressure on the nerve. This, of course, is accompanied by pain in all the areas which the nerve innervates.

Dan's Pain - A Case Study

Dan, a 45-year-old man, appeared in my office complaining of low back pain radiating down the entire length of his left leg. The leg pain began a week before he came to the clinic. He said he had suffered from low back pain in recent months, but after bending down to pick up a pen that had fallen from his desk, he felt a sharp, sudden pain that radiated down his left leg, accompanied by numbness and a loss of feeling in the outer leg and the small toe of his left foot.

He told me that since then, although he had taken medication, the pain had been very bad and he could not obtain relief. It was especially aggravating when he sat down, coughed and when putting on his socks or pants. Dan, his whole body bent towards the right, claimed he was very tired and unable to sleep at night because of the pain, and said that even when he managed to fall asleep for a few hours, he would awaken with cramps in the gastrocnemius muscle at the back of his left leg. He did not complain of any other symptoms. A CT scan performed two days prior to his appointment with me showed a left L5-S1 disc herniation, accompanied by nerve pressure on the root of nerve S1 on the left.

Dan came to my clinic for treatment following recommendations from friends. I gave him medical treatments, along with guidance on how to carry out various activities in his home in order to minimize the possibility of his condition deteriorating and to accelerate the recovery process. The counseling included, among other things, specific exercises for his condition, instructions on how to bend correctly, how to put on shoes and socks despite his acute pain, how to cough in a way that will not hurt, and how to get into the car and into bed with minimal pain.

Dan's improvement was rapid. First, the pain in his leg decreased significantly and the cramps in the leg muscles ceased. This finally allowed him to sleep better at night. His lower back pain also improved, but at a slower pace. After a few days, Dan reported that the feeling in his leg was much better and that he felt little pain in his back. Dan was now able to stand up straight without tilting to the right.

We continued to work together in the treatment program that I had set for him, and Dan soon returned to normal function at home and at work. He continued to follow the instructions I gave him to maintain his condition and to prevent, as much as possible, the emergence of new problems. Dan has since continued with preventive treatments for his back and spine.

•••

How to Put Shoes on and Tie Laces, Even When Suffering from a Protruding or Herniated Disc?

Putting on and lacing shoes are two examples of the most difficult actions for those who suffer from lumbar disc protrusion or a herniated disc. This is especially true in the morning, shortly after waking up. Early in the morning, after a night's sleep or following a midday rest, the body is inflexible which makes it difficult to perform these actions. Therefore it is advised to "warm up" the body a little beforehand, for example by walking around the house for a few minutes, and even perform at least one flexibility exercise for the lower back.

The main mistake made by those suffering from disc problems, especially in the acute stage accompanied by severe pain, is an attempt to put on shoes while sitting. This entails the person bending and arching the back. Bending the torso while sitting causes increased pressure on the discs **and can worsen the condition and delay healing.**

Therefore, do not sit down to put your shoes on or tie laces while sitting, and refrain from bending your back.

One way to perform these tasks is to crouch down, buttocks touching your heels and your lower back in a lordotic position (concaved arch shape). Bring one foot forward and place it on the floor. Now, lower the opposite knee to the floor. Lean forward, keeping your back straight, and perform the task. See Figure 32 below. After doing so, do the same with the other foot. When you want to get up, return to a squatting position and stand up, again keeping your back straight, using your leg muscles to help you stand.

Another option, although less convenient, is to stand in front of a chair, as close as possible. Put one foot on the chair, with your knee bent at about 90 degrees, bend the knee of the leg standing on the floor, lean forward keeping your back straight and perform the task. See Figure 33 below. Once you have finished, switch legs and tie the next shoe.

If these methods are difficult to perform, you can always seek the help of another person.

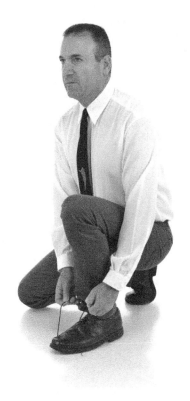

Figure 32: Tying Laces - Option A

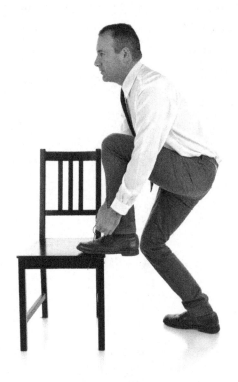

Figure 33: Tying Laces - Option B

Recommended Seats During a Flight for Those Suffering from a Protruding or Herniated Disc

Many people plan their annual vacation a long time in advance, flying to a destination they have dreamed of for a long time. Then suddenly ... they slip a disc and suffer from acute pain. Despite this, there is no way they are going to give up on their vacation, and all they want is to safely get through the flight. In contrast to travelling in a car or bus where you can stop and get out of the vehicle to stretch your legs and continue the journey as you please, this is not possible on a plane, and even your freedom of movement is restricted. Sitting on a plane is also less convenient than in a vehicle; it is more crowded, the journey is of a longer duration, and with less legroom and minimal options for adjusting the seat.

If you are a person who already suffers from a disc problem, flying is even more difficult, and your main concern will be how to survive sitting down for so long. When purchasing your airline ticket, try to find a seat where you can get up as often as possible and where you can do some exercises, while causing minimum disturbance to other passengers and crew.

Obviously, a window seat or sitting in the middle of the row is not a good choice since you will have to disturb other passengers every time you wish to leave your seat. What if the person sitting next to you has fallen asleep? Do you wake them up or suffer in silence?

Therefore, it is better to choose to sit in an aisle seat where you can get up whenever you like without having to disturb other passengers. A better option is to pick an aisle seat towards the **back of the plane** where you can get up and perform some stretching exercises without worrying about other passengers watching you and without disturbing the crew. Usually these seats are close to the toilet, which is another good reason for a person with disc problems to choose them, as sometimes frequent urination can occur for someone with a herniated disc.

How to Get Into Bed Without Pain?

Many patients who visit my clinic and who suffer acute pain find it problematic to get on the treatment bed and wonder how they will manage to get into bed at home. Due to acute pain, sitting is out of the question, while standing and walking can also be a tiring task. All they want is to rest their back a little and reduce their acute pain.

Most people who do not suffer from back pain bend their backs and spine when getting into bed. However, if someone suffers from acute low back pain due to disc herniation, whether the pain radiates down the leg or not, such a movement as bending the body and back can cause acute pain. Therefore, one of their biggest challenges may be to get into bed without bending their back and without sitting. While they may suffer severe pains when climbing into bed, even if they change their habits as described below, it is advisable for them to perform gentle and slow backward movements of the lower back while standing, before actually getting into bed.

In my experience with many patients, getting into bed, after performing these backward arching exercises, becomes easier.

It is Time To Practice!

1. Stand next to your bed, legs slightly apart and try to keep your back as straight as you can.
2. Rotate your body slightly so that your head is facing the head of the bed.

3. Bend the knee of your leg that is closest to the head of bed and place your hand (on the same side of your body) on the bed.

4. Move your weight forward towards the bed and place the other hand similarly on the bed. Make sure you do not bend your back and keep your head in line.

5. Lift the other leg as straight as possible onto the bed, lower your pelvis onto the bed and raise the other leg.

6. Now, bend your elbows and try to lean on them for 10 to 15 seconds. If this is hard for you, move your hands to the side of your body.

That's it! You have managed to get into bed! If you want to turn around, do it in one movement without bending your back.

Traction or Compression? Methods for Treating Problematic Discs

There are many treatment methods and techniques for dealing with a problematic disc. Only after conducting a thorough examination of the patient, taking into account his overall state of health, can the therapist decide on the best course of treatment.

Common treatment methods combine a series of **traction** or **compression** exercises. The idea of traction is to separate the vertebrae from each other, which creates a space for the disc to move and slip back towards its original position (although it may not reach the actual original position). The separation of the vertebrae increases the gap that the spinal nerve passes through, and thus there is less nerve pressure. Other techniques attempt to compress the disc back towards into its normal place, thereby distancing it from the root of the nerve and reducing the pain.

In many cases, bending the lower back forward causes the disc to protrude or slip backwards out of place. Using a compression technique such as the one applied while extending and arching backwards the lower back, which is the reverse of the injury mechanism, can lead to a rapid recovery.

Again, I would like to emphasize that there are many methods of treatment for disc problems, and it is necessary to consult with a professional and receive medical advice.

Lying Down

How to Reduce and Prevent Back Pain While Lying Down?

Many people experience less back pain during the day, while in motion, than in bed at night. As evening approaches, their minds start to wander with the thought of maybe suffering another night of pain and lack of sleep, causing them to function poorly during the day and experience fatigue.

Back and neck pain felt while lying down can stem from a variety of reasons. For example, inflammation of the vertebrae, trauma from falling, a fracture or any other injury, oncological vertebral problems, problems in ribs attached to the vertebrae, problems in pelvic bones, Scoliosis and advanced degenerative changes of the vertebrae can all cause back and neck pain.

During many years of treating patients in my clinic, one of the most common causes of back and neck pain which I have encountered is related to problems with the intervertebral disc, especially due to a protruding or herniated disc. Cervical disc herniation or a protruding disc in this area can cause pain in the neck and arm, sometimes accompanied by a numbness or 'shooting pains' that radiate down the arm while in a lying position. Disc problems in the lower back, may cause similar symptoms in the lower back and leg when lying down.

During the day when we move, the muscles of the legs, pelvis, back, and abdomen absorb shocks, and together with the joints of the vertebrae and pelvis, reduce the burden on the intervertebral disc. At night, while lying down, these muscles and joints are at rest and are not weight bearing. At the same time, the discs absorb fluid from the surrounding area, causing them to expand and swell slightly. The same problematic disc, whether protruding or herniated, slightly changes shape when our body rests in a horizontal position. This causes greater pressure to be exerted on the nerves, resulting in numbness, pain, 'shooting pains' in the limbs, etc.

One of the therapeutic methods which helps many patients who come to my clinic with disc problems and pain during the night, is to implement correct exercise during the day! It amazes me every time I see people who have suffered from weeks of pain and sleepless nights, follow my instructions and suddenly succeed in finally getting a good night's sleep! The more correct actions we take with our backs during the day, the more comfortable sleep will be at night, as well as getting up in the morning. Specific spinal treatments and exercises, along with optimal body behavior in the simplest of actions such as washing your face, entering and exiting a vehicle, putting on socks and shoes, lifting things, etc., can help improve your quality of sleep.

It is essential, of course, to seek appropriate medical consultation in order to speed up the recovery process and improve the quality of sleep.

Nightly pain improvement is usually gradual. For example, if at first the person suffering had a habit of waking up at one o'clock in the morning because of the pain, and the night after awoke at two-thirty and the night after that woke up at four in the morning, this proves that the patient managed to gradually sleep longer, which is an excellent sign of his progress. The longer the duration of sleep, the more proof they are on the right path to recovery.

During sleep itself, it is more difficult to perform actions to reduce pain, and in some cases, we do not have good control over our bodies while lying down. A person may fall asleep on his back and during the night, toss and turn in different directions, and wake up in the morning to find himself laying in the same position he fell asleep.

He might think that he lay on his back all night without moving, but of course that is not the case.

In terms of sleeping positions, lying on one's stomach is not recommended. This position causes the head to move to one side in order to breathe, creating asymmetry along the length of the neck muscles and shoulder blades, between the right side and left. This can cause pain, especially in the neck and shoulders, and an asymmetrical stretching of the back muscles, as well as causing a long-term approximation of the lumbar vertebrae, thus increasing the risk of lower back pain. Back pain worsens when people who prefer to lay on their stomach place a pillow under their heads.

Lying on your back can relieve back and neck pain. However, if you lie on your back and lay your head on several pillows, causing the upper part of your body to be significantly higher than the lower part, pain in the neck or lower back can actually worsen. If you do not suffer from dizziness or breathing problems, consider lowering the height of the pillows.

Those suffering from lower back pain at night sometimes find relief in bending the knees and thighs while lying sideways, otherwise known as the fetal position.

Lying on the side at night can also give relief to those suffering from spinal pain which radiates to the hands or legs. Many people suffering this kind of pain will find relief by lying sideways, with the painful limb in the uppermost position and the other resting on the bed. When lying down in this position, it is advisable that the head be in line with the spine and placed on a pillow which is neither too high nor too low.

The mattress also plays an important part in the quality of your sleep. It should be adapted to your body structure and the condition of your vertebrae. You should consider occasionally turning the mattress, if possible.

Sometimes you can decide to lie in bed longer than you are normally accustomed. Prolonged lying down or sleep may increase pain, especially towards the morning or when getting up.

Secrets from the Bedroom

Many people suffer from lower back pain and their quality of life is impaired. Sometimes a seemingly simple movement causes them great suffering and their fear is that another simple similar action can cause additional harm. Many people ask for my advice on how to improve their day-to-day functioning, and prevent pain and aggravation.

"Doctor, is Sex Out of the Question?" A Case Study

One day I received an email from one of my patients with a personal question. "Doctor, is sex out of the question?" he asked. My reply to him was that you have to enjoy life.

In my opinion, life is not based on black or white, and yes or no. Life is made up of many other shades of color; that is, I believe in an optimistic approach and in performing actions that make us feel pleasure, **but with forethought.**

Following a series of medical treatments, the above-mentioned patient's back had improved considerably, his lower back movement was almost fully restored, and he was pain free. There was no apparent reason to a limited sex life. However, since his initial complaint before he began treatment was back pain that worsened when bending his back, I recommended that he perform several backward arching exercises before he get into bed.

●●●

Nevertheless, what happens when someone suffers with low back pain and still craves sexual activity? Are there certain positions that can aggravate the problem he suffers from? Are there positions that make things easier for those who have lumbar disc problems?

As I mentioned in the previous chapters, one must be aware of the various situations in which pain appears. For example, many people suffer from back pain due to various disc problems. Therefore, a sitting position or one that simulates sitting can exacerbate their pain.

Lying on your back when your upper torso is much higher-positioned in comparison to your lower body (,for example, with a number of pillows under your head,) can also aggravate pain. In general, people who suffer from pain while sitting in a slouched position, and not upright, should refrain from arching or bending forward the lower back in the various sex positions, which could worsen their pain.

And vice versa, if a backward movement of the back causes pain, such as movements that emphasize and slightly deepen the lumbar arch, it is best to avoid various intimate positions which exaggerate this. These people will often find relief in other positions which do not involve a backward movement.

If you would like to learn more on this topic, you should read the new and groundbreaking study conducted by Professor Stuart McGill and Natalie Sidorkewicz of Waterloo Ontario University, Canada.[2]

---

2   McGill, S. Sidorkewicz, N. (2014) Male Spine Motion During Coitus. Implications for the Low Back Pain Patient, Spine: 39 (20) . Sep 1633-9. doi:10.1097/BRS.0000000000000518.
McGill, S. Sidorkewicz, N. (2015) Documenting Female Spine Motion During Coitus with a Commentary on the Implications for the Low Back Pain Patient: Eur Spine J. Mar;24(3):513-20. doi: 10.1007/s00586-014-3626-y.

The Effect of Obesity on Back Pain

One of the most troublesome problems today is the problem of obesity. This condition results in an increase in body fat, causes functional problems and many diseases. Obesity can increase the likelihood of heart problems such as hypertension, diabetes, cerebral events, cancers such as bowel cancer, as well as increased stress on joints such as hip and knee joints. Obesity can affect and make motion more difficult, causing lack of movement, which leads to weight gain and acceleration of degenerative processes in back and legs joints, along with weakening muscles in these areas.

Fat in the abdomen tends to accumulate around the internal organs and causes the abdomen to protrude and droop. This shifts the body's center of gravity forward, and in order to not fall forward, the muscles in the back need to work much harder. In this situation, additional pressure placed on the intervertebral discs may lead to an increase in the risk of future injuries to the back muscles and discs.

As more fat accumulates in the abdominal area, more pressure is applied to the anatomical structures in the back, increasing the risk of damage. Therefore, it is advisable to remain within normal weight range. Abdominal fat pushes and stretches the abdominal muscles forward and causes their elongation, making the pelvis less stable and causing a forward rotation of the pelvis.

This causes more weight load on back muscles, ligaments, tendons and discs, causes vertebral misalignment and increases the rate of degenerative processes in the vertebral joints. It can also increase the lumbar curve thus compressing the vertebrae so they are closer to each other.

Therefore, correct guided nutrition and exercise are advisable in order to combat the negative effects of obesity.

The Effect Coughing or Sneezing Has on Pain Levels

Coughing and sneezing are very common and natural reflexes. Colds, flu, asthma, smoking and various problems in the respiratory system can all cause coughing. Sneezing often originates from viral infections in the respiratory tract and various allergens in the air. Although these common actions seem simple, they may cause damage to the back, and many people have noted a feeling of pain in the lower back, or even in the middle of the back and between the shoulder blades, while coughing or sneezing.

Coughing and sneezing is the result of pressure, built up inside the body, looking for an 'escape route'. When the pressure exits the body, by coughing or sneezing, it can cause a quick, sudden and sharp forward bend in the body and spine, which can cause muscle pain.

In addition, coughing and sneezing can increase pressure on the intervertebral disc, so the condition of the disc can deteriorate. Cervical disc deterioration due to coughing or sneezing can cause complaints of pain and numbness in the hands, as well as headaches. Involvement of the lumbar disc after coughing or sneezing can lead to various complaints of leg pain, 'shooting pain' down the leg, etc.

In order to prevent back pain and reduce existing pain, it is advisable to take several steps before or during coughing or sneezing.

1. **Standing.** Try to avoid coughing or sneezing while sitting; preferably **get up from the chair** and perform these actions in a standing position.

2. **Backward Arching of the Back.** If you are unable to get up from the chair while coughing or sneezing, it is advisable to slightly arch your lower back backwards, and avoid bending your lower back and neck forwards while sitting.

3. **Support.** While standing, you can support your lower back with one hand while laying the other on a table. By slightly bending your knees and refraining from bending your back forwards, the chance of lower back and neck damage decrease.

Sometimes, due to illness, people are bedridden. They often lie on their backs with their upper torso positioned higher than their feet and with several pillows to support their head. Again, the spine is in a bent position and frequent coughing and sneezing can exacerbate spinal problems. Lying on the side can minimize the risk of back pain.

These slight changes in posture can prevent greater damage in the future.

Sporting Activities

How to Maintain Strong Back Vertebrae?

Osteoporosis is one of the most common diseases which affects skeletal and spinal bones. This disease, although most common in women, can also affect men, causes a decrease in bone density and strength, thus increasing the risk of bone and vertebrae fractures. Therefore, maintaining proper nutrition, and reducing smoking and alcohol consumption is very important from an early age in order to maintain stronger bones later in life.

Physical activity and proper posture have significant emphasis on preventing osteoporosis. These activities are advisable for any age and it is never too late to start! Many people sit in a slouched position for many hours both at work and at home. They do not engage in physical activity in which the body is in a vertical position, for instance, walking, climbing stairs instead of using the elevator, dancing, etc. Therefore, the strength of the bones in the legs, pelvis and vertebrae decreases, and the chances of future problems arise. The osteoporotic vertebrae lose their strength, their density decreases - much like a sponge with many holes - and therefore can only withstand lighter weight loads.

The vertebrae gradually weaken and can change their shape and position. Poor, forward, and slouched posture, common to many, along with the gradual weakening of the vertebrae, can lead to compression of the frontal part of the vertebral body and possible compression fractures of the vertebrae. The vertebrae, then, is compressed and changes shape, and instead of resembling a square-shape, forms a trapezoidal or wedge-like shape, creating a chain reaction to the rest of the spine and causing it to bend even more. This bending of the vertebrae, the result of weak vertebrae, causes back pain and greater pressure and functional disorders of internal organs such as the heart and lungs.

Some of my patients suffer from osteoporosis, and their chance of fracture, especially in one of the lower thoracic vertebrae or in one of the upper lumbar vertebrae, is increased. Sometimes even bending and lifting a light object can result in a vertebral fracture, and it does not necessarily have to be traumatic!

I advise my patients to regularly exercise, maintain good posture, and perform specific exercises for their spine and back. Prolonged exercises which include bending the back and vertebrae, such as sitting and trying to touch your ankles with your hands, for example, are tricky exercises that can accelerate the deterioration of the vertebra leading to an osteoporotic fracture. Alternatively, I recommend various back exercises that can be performed while lying on your stomach or hands and knees, which contribute to strengthening and maintaining the natural lumbar curve. See Figure 34 below. These exercises are very important to strengthen the back, improve posture and reduce pain, even if you already suffer from osteoporosis.

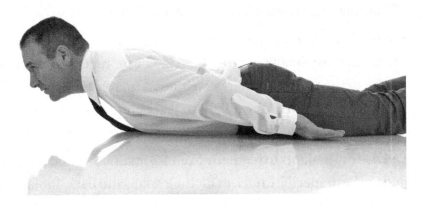

Figure 34: Raising the upper torso to strengthen the back

Optimal Spinal Motion Range

Motion is one of the human body's most important functions and without it, our quality of life would be very poor. Imagine what the consequences to our health would be if the blood in our bodies passed through the blood vessels too slowly or in an insufficient quantity. So too, are correct body and spinal movements necessary to maintain optimal health. Spinal movements in different directions allow us to perform tasks and daily activities in a more convenient way. The more limited the movements of the spine, the more difficult it will be to perform actions. Prolonged restriction of movement in the neck, back or pelvis is usually associated with degenerative changes in the same area where the movement restriction exists.

The spine should be able to move in six directions: to bend forward and backward, bend left and right, and rotate left and right. Many people suffer from movement restriction of the back and neck in one or more of the directions indicated above, which is one of the important signs of a back and/or neck problem. In some cases, pain will be felt in addition to a limitation of movement, and in some cases there will be no pain at all.

Those who suffer movement restriction accompanied by pain are those who seek medical consultation. On the other hand, many who do not feel pain are unaware of both the limitation and the negative consequences that movement impairment can cause.

Limited back and neck movement can be due to a variety of reasons. The most common ones are associated with chronic or acute muscle problems such as muscle contraction or shortened muscles. Sometimes movement restriction is due to degeneration of the vertebral joints or inadequate movement of the vertebrae, similar to a machine in a factory with rusty wheels that is difficult to operate, and sometimes it is due to intervertebral disc problems such as a protruding or herniated disc. These symptoms cause a person to bend sideways or forward, and they will find difficulty in standing straight.

A combination of normal muscle length, freely moving joints and well functioning discs located in optimal positions will all contribute in achieving normal spinal movement.

One of the most significant ranges that is frequently overlooked is the backward motion of the spine and backward-diagonal movements. For most of our lives we sit for too many hours at home, at work and in the car, therefore the head, neck, shoulders, lower back, and pelvis are already in a state of flexion. Even in a slouched sitting position, common to many, our body and spine bend forward. When we sit, doze or fall asleep in an armchair, our head and upper torso, from the pelvis up, falls and bends forward and downwards rather than backward. Add to that the slow, gradual wear-and-tear process of the spine which makes us look bent as we age, and you have a whole range of behaviors that affect our posture.

When do we implement backward motion of the torso? Few people maintain correct spine mobility when stretching backward. See Figure 35 below. Therefore, it is no wonder that many suffer from back pain, degeneration of the joints and disc herniation! These actions should be performed at the right frequency, at the right speed and with correct posture. Perseverance in maintaining the natural curves of the spine, and especially the backward motion, even if we do not have back pain, can save us a lot of damage.

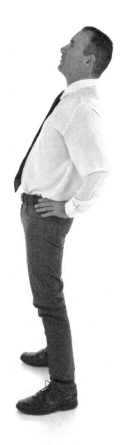

Figure 35: Maintaining spinal mobility through backward stretches

188 | Dr. Ronen Welgrin

Learn the Importance
of Abdominal Muscles

The stomach is a part of body that bothers many people. Complaints such as "I am too fat," "My belly is sticking out," "I cannot get rid of my stomach, and if I could only lose my stomach, my back would hurt less," are all commonly heard. The desire to address this problem is great, but not many know how to go about it.

Abdominal muscles play great importance in general body health due to their location, the way they are deployed, how they function and their points of contact with the body. The abdominal muscles consist of several layers and act in different directions. They connect the pelvic bones to the chest and ribs, providing them great strength and the opportunity to maintain and protect internal organs. For example, the heart, lungs and liver are protected by the ribs, but what protects abdominal organs such as the uterus, intestines and other organs?

The abdominal muscles create a frontal wall to protect internal organs, and the weakness of the abdominal muscles can create a bulging and protruding belly. A forward fall of the abdomen causes organs to move out of place, pressure on blood vessels, and, of course, more stress on the lower back. The abdominal muscles are also connected to the ribs, so they are auxiliary muscles in breathing and prevent the movement of the thoracic cage from its natural position.

Most people have the desire and ambition to strengthen their abdominal muscles, however those who exercise can make a number of mistakes while seeking to strengthen the abdominal muscles, which can damage the spine and back.

1. **Preparation and warm up exercises.** Sometimes, those who exercise begin to strengthen the abdominal muscles without prior preparation. For example, when people who work in front of a computer suddenly decide to get up from their chair, lie down on the floor and begin abdomen strengthening exercises, this sudden movement without warm up exercises can increase the chance of injury. Therefore, it is recommended to walk for at least a few minutes to improve cardiovascular endurance and perform flexibility exercises and general joint movement before any such activity.

2. **First and foremost...back muscles.** People who exercise tend to skip stretching lower back muscles before strengthening the abdominal muscles. Therefore, it is recommended to lie on your back, cross your feet on a mattress, and hold each knee one at a time, close to the chest for 20 seconds. It is best to repeat this exercise several times on each side, and then hold both knees together, close to the chest, for a similar length of time and repeat this exercise several times. See Figure 36 below. By stretching the lower back muscles, the effectiveness of strengthening abdominal muscles will be better, thereby reducing the likelihood of back injuries that may occur in muscles, ligaments or discs.

3. **Do not elevate your torso too high!** Elevating your upper torso too high from a laying down position can cause back damage. The maximum upward movement should be until the shoulder blades do not touch the floor. Beyond that, the

iliopsoas muscle in the pelvis becomes involved in the action, and this may cause compression of the lumbar vertebrae. See Figure 37 below. Excessive elevation of the torso will cause the back to arch and bend. This, combined with compression of the vertebrae and discs due to iliopsoas muscular activity, can result in damage to the ligaments and discs in the back.

4. **Head support**. Pull your head and neck up with your hands instead of just supporting the head in your palms. In the same elevating position described above, the palms are placed behind the head. Many, instead of using the abdominal muscles to lift the upper torso, use the palms to lift the head. This causes the cervical spine to stretch and bend during elevation, which can lead to possible muscle, vertebrae and disc damage of the neck. Another option is to hold your hands over your ears instead of pulling your neck with your hands, thus saving neck damage. See Figure 38 below.

Consulting with a professional is always advisable before deciding to strengthen your abdominal muscles.

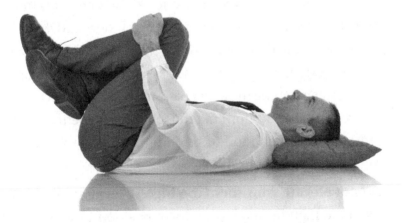

Figure 36: Holding both knees close to the chest to extend and elongate the back muscles

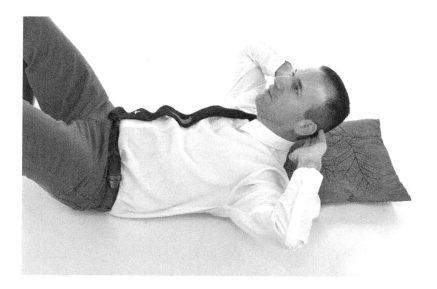

Figure 37: Elevation of the upper torso until the shoulder blades are not touching the floor, in order to strengthen the abdominal muscles and prevent damage to the back

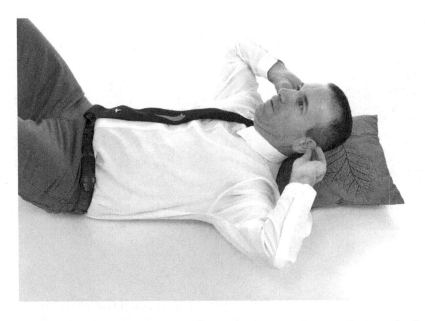

Figure 38: Placing your fingers over your ears instead of pulling the neck with your hands to avoid neck damage

Know How to Strengthen Your Back Muscles

Whether you are suffering from back pain or not, strengthening the back muscles plays an extremely important role in maintaining your health. We use back muscles in many different body actions such as walking, swimming, dancing, getting up from a chair, entering and exiting a vehicle, cleaning the house and many more daily activities.

The natural inclination of our bodies is to lean forward. If we fall asleep sitting down, we will find that our heads sag downward and our bodies collapse and tilt forward. In the common aging process of the body and spine, the back bends forwards. Back muscles are a very important factor in our posture and, among other things, help prevent the head and the rest of the body from falling forward and downwards.

We have more than 100 muscles on or attached to our back, and although we think, that this great muscular system will protect us, that is not the case. Many people who visit my clinic suffer from back and muscle pain, and they are not even aware that their back muscles are not at their best. The muscles are arranged in several layers, at different degrees of depth, in different directions, in different lengths, emerge and attach to different places in the back, with each muscle responsible for a different action and function. Therefore, it is important to strengthen and stretch them in a variety of ways.

For example, sometimes it is necessary to strengthen these muscles in a slow and controlled manner, and sometimes we need to do it rapidly. Sometimes these muscles need to be strengthened over for a short period, and sometimes they need a longer strengthening period. Sometimes they need to be operated in a partial range of motion, and sometimes will need a greater range of motion to strengthen them. Sometimes doing back exercises against our own body weight is enough and sometimes, additional weight will be needed to add resistance. Sometimes muscles need to act in a static way, and sometimes in a dynamic way.

Strong back muscles can, among other things, reduce existing pain, prevent new problems, improve your posture and quality of life, improve your self image and effectively absorb more loads and shocks, which would otherwise penetrate softer tissues such as a disc or a ligament and cause damage.

The Connection between Cellular Phones and Back Weakness in Children

Back pain problems are often associated with a lack of or neglect of the strengthening of the back muscles. Every year, the age of patients who visit my clinic gets younger and younger. One of the main reasons for this is children's increasing use of cellular phones and other mobile devices. Prolonged use of such devices elongates and weakens the child's back muscles, exposing them to continuous damage. Children usually sit for long hours while bending their necks and backs, which can cause them great harm later in life and they usually do not relate their pain to the excessive use of the cellular device.

During one of my lectures to fifth and sixth grade students on correct posture and how to prevent back problems, I asked the students to lie on their stomachs and perform various exercises while holding their cellular phones.

In one of the exercises, I asked the students to send a text message to their classmates while they were lying on their stomachs, without their elbows and hands touching the floor! This exercise made them use and strengthen their back muscles.

I explained to them that this is the **proper position** we are supposed to keep during the day (maintaining the inward lumbar curve), but since most tend to lean forward while typing text messages ,the inward lumbar curve is not maintained, the back weakens, resulting in damage over time.

Although at the end of the exercise, the children understood the need to look after and maintain their backs, I am confident that a single lecture did not adequately emphasize the importance in back protection amongst children and youth. Educational frameworks are currently lacking in providing continuous and consistent education regarding the importance of correct posture and how to maintain a healthy back. Unfortunately, most parents also do not understand the importance of this subject.

As always, I recommend that you seek professional medical consultation on how to strengthen your back muscles, keeping in mind your general health.

Learn How to Strengthen Your Leg Muscles to Avoid Back Pain

Considerable back damage can be prevented by proper and correct use of the leg muscles. Common actions such as lifting objects, moving from lying to sitting and from sitting to standing, engaging in sports activities, etc. should all be implemented with proper and correct movements of the legs. This will ensure that the leg muscles will absorb the weight load thereby reducing pressure on the back and spine. This requires, among other things, regular strengthening of the leg muscles.

Even people who work in a prolonged sitting position need to know how to strengthen their leg muscles. If you work out in a gym, you will need to know which devices and which body positions are the best for strengthening leg muscles, which positions exert a large load on the vertebrae and discs, and which positions exert less.

Many people become aware of the importance of strengthening leg muscles when their backs are in an acute state. In this situation, acute back pain makes it very difficult to perform any simple action and people are forced to carry them out with the help of the leg muscles. Nevertheless, because their leg muscles are not strong enough, they continue to perform these actions with their backs in an incorrect manner, thus delaying the healing process.

Strengthening the leg muscles may be performed at any age and anywhere, and, if performed correctly and regularly, can help prevent back problems.

198 | Dr. Ronen Welgrin

Epilogue

I hope that you enjoyed and will benefit from reading this book. I strongly believe that adhering to the guidelines and insights described in the book will provide you with a solid, practical basis for understanding how to reduce, prevent and even eliminate back and spinal pain.

We have read about the crucial importance of the spine and the spinal nerves that reach all parts of the body. We have learned that the spine cannot be replaced, and therefore must be protected from the many dangers lurking in our lives. We now understand that correct body conduct while standing, sitting, lifting objects and lying down are very significant in order to maintain and enable the proper functioning of the spine.

I encourage you to continue to enrich your knowledge on this subject, to consult with physicians, therapists and other health care professionals.

I hope that paying continuous attention to correct behavior patterns and daily actions related to the spine as described in this book will lead you to live well and enjoy a good quality of life.

Furthermore, I will be happy to help you with any questions you may have in order to help improve your well-being.

Wishing you a healthy life,
Dr. Ronen Welgrin, D.C.

Made in the USA
Coppell, TX
29 February 2020